THE
LEAN BODY
MANUAL

THE
LEAN BODY
MANUAL

Jon Pearlman

EVOLVE

PUBLISHING HOUSE

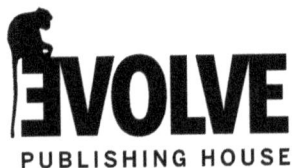

An Evolve Publishing House Book
This edition first published in 2017, by Evolve Publishing House, LLC,
Florida, United States of America.

Cover design by Alex "Ex" Makarov
Cover photos by Lara Rose
Book design by Marijo Šarić

The information provided here is intended to assist you in making informed choices about your body, health, and fitness. This book is intended to supplement, not replace, proper exercise training. The author and publisher advise that readers be fully responsible for their safety and understand their limitations. Before performing the workout routines provided, be sure that your equipment is well-maintained, and do not overstep your experience level, aptitude, and physical condition. The recommendations for exercise and specific foods in this book are not intended to replace medical advice, care, or any exercise routine or dietary regimen that may have been prescribed by your doctor. Like with all exercise and dietary recommendations, you should get your doctor's approval before starting.

Mention of specific products, companies, organizations, or authorities in this book does not imply endorsement by the author or publisher; nor does mention of specific companies, organizations, or authorities in the book imply that they endorse this book. The author and the publisher disclaim any liability or loss, personal or otherwise, resulting from the recommendations and procedures of this program.

For more information, please visit www.MissionLean.com.

Library of Congrss Cataloging-in-Publication Data
Library of Congress Control Number: 2017906428
Name: Pearlman, Jon, 1988— author.
Title: The Lean Body Manual / Jon Pearlman.
Description: Florida : Evolve Publishing House, LLC, [2017]
Website: www.MissionLean.com
Identifiers: ISBN 978-0-9907859-2-7 (paperback)
              ISBN 978-0-9907859-3-4 (e-book)
Subjects: LCSH: Physical Fitness (sh85101540)
                 Nutrition (sh85093451)
                 Health (sh85059518)
Classification: DDC : 613/.7
p. cm.

Table of Contents

Part IV: The Lean Body Fitness Program

Part V: The Lean Body Meal Plan

Testimonials

Acknowledgements

About the Author

Introduction:

My name is Jon Pearlman and I have dedicated my life to building the lean, athletic body.

In the pages to come, I will outline my unique framework for optimizing fitness, nutrition, and lifestyle—so that you can achieve your peak form. I will present you with countless tricks and tips, and realizations I've learned along the way that will skyrocket you into the best shape of your life.

This book is a hands-on guide and manual for those who aspire to build the lean body. Part I, "Build the V-12 Body," addresses how to best approach your daily fitness routines so that you can maximize your physical training. Part II, "Perfect Your Nutrition," outlines a feasible and sustainable path to eating healthfully, so that your body is optimally fueled and you're living life energized, satiated, and free of cravings. Part III, "Lean Down Your Life," presents strategies for getting the most out of your lean body efforts. Part IV, "The Lean Body Fitness Program" outlines all of the fitness exercises you will need to build the lean body, along with a 4-week jump-starter program to get you on your way. Part V, "The Lean Body Meal Plan," provides you with the grocery list and recipes that will allow you to lean down, along with a 4-week meal plan so you can start shedding the excess weight immediately.

All of these components—exercise, nutrition, lifestyle, and a clear-cut plan of action—feed off of one another to produce the desired result.

Failing to tackle one of them will prevent you from succeeding in the others. Perfecting your approach to fitness and diet is a formula that combines inputs on multiple planes to produce a three-dimensional product: The Lean Body. You're in luck because my lean body approach is highly effective and it will get you the results you want...not just for the short-term, but for many years to come.

No more time to waste. Let's start getting lean.

PART I:
BUILD THE
V-12 BODY

CHAPTER 1
GET LEAN

Turn Your Body into the V-12

Getting lean comes with many great benefits along the way. If you master your physical routines, you're going to feel and look great. If you're taking care of your body, you'll be healthy and invigorated.

Everyone can appreciate a top-end sports car, and having lived in South Florida for the past several years, I often see a Ferrari, Lamborghini, or Bugatti driving by, or parked in front of a fancy restaurant. The reality is, though, you don't need millions of dollars to own a V-12. If you perfect your fitness and nutrition routines, you can start building a V-12...*in your own body*! Constructing a finely-tuned, functional, healthy, enduring, lean, sleek, toned, strong, powerful, robust, limber, quick, agile, and flexible body should be your goal—and this is what *The Lean Body Manual* is all about.

The work required to convert your body into a V-12 may very well be comparable in volume to the work necessary to purchase one in automobile form. But I'm pretty sure you can guess which of these V-12s contains more value.

Reaching the V-12 body will take time and resolve. Yet if you're committed, you will surely prevail. You just need to stay focused, adjust your lifestyle, and keep pushing until you arrive.

Why Lean?

The lean body is the most difficult physique to build because the workout plan revolves around *cardiovascular* conditioning. At the end of the day, there's nothing harder than raising your heart-rate, keeping it elevated, and sweating. You will need to get used to this type of workout if you aren't accustomed to it, but overcoming the initial hurdles will be necessary to get to your final destination. With persistence, you will achieve a lean, functional, athletic, and *enduring* physique.

The "get big/get jacked" mindset has become mainstream in fitness—espeically for men. Instead of playing sports, running, and building lean and functional muscle, the majority of people are lifting heavy weights and looking to get huge. The problem is that the body-building workouts that create large peripheral muscles fail to work the most important muscle of all: the heart.

This new-age weight-lifting craze is just a smart way to get you to buy more product: protein shakes, supplements, pills, powders, energy drinks, diet plans, workout books, exercise classes, gym memberships, etc. Sorting through this mess is nearly impossible, and with a heavy enough weight or sufficiently complicated exercise move, you'll soon get injured and need to spend more money in the form of healthcare services: doctors' visits, physical therapy, pain killers, chiropractic adjustments, homeopathic remedies, surgeries, "KT" tape, braces, "sleeves," and the list goes on. Getting lean and staying healthy is simple if you train in the right way. You just need to have your wits about you so you can circumvent the noise and propaganda.

As you begin to make headway through this book, you'll soon realize that most of what's out there is preventing you from reaching top form, and not only that, but it's making you poorer in the process! Your own willpower, dedication, persistence, and body is what's going to get you there.

Once you begin asking the right questions and working with your body in a targeted way—in the *correct* way—you'll soon foster clarity and accelerate your transition towards the V-12 body. We can all represent this new era of fitness together—an era based in health, longevity, and logic—one grounded in the lean, athletic body.

Become an Athlete

The lean body is both functional and enduring.

"Functional" means that the muscles and tendons of your body can work in unison, for some physiological purpose—running, let's say, or playing a sport. Body weight exercises and cardiovascular training form the basis for building the functional body, and the full training routines that you should follow are provided in Part IV of the book.

An "enduring" body means that you've built muscles that will last a lifetime—something that body-building doesn't facilitate. Large, bulky muscles convert to fat rapidly if you don't work them out continuously. Those who follow the path of heavy weight-lifting usually experience ups and downs frequently—these people will look completely ripped one month, and then tubby the next. That's also why you often see extreme "before" and "after" pictures in magazines and supplement advertisements of people following a weight-based training program—such individuals might very well have undergone *many* of these "transformations" over the course of their lives. In contrast, once you build the lean body, you will have it for life. Taking a break from your training won't result in any significant weight gain or muscle loss.

If you have a background as an athlete, you must use the sport you play to assist you in your pursuit of the lean body. Your sport should be the foundation of your functional training. If you were a competitive track athlete or swimmer, stick to your training routines to the best of your ability even though your competitive career may have ended. If you're a tennis or soccer player, find games on the weekends so you can keep your athletic edge intact.

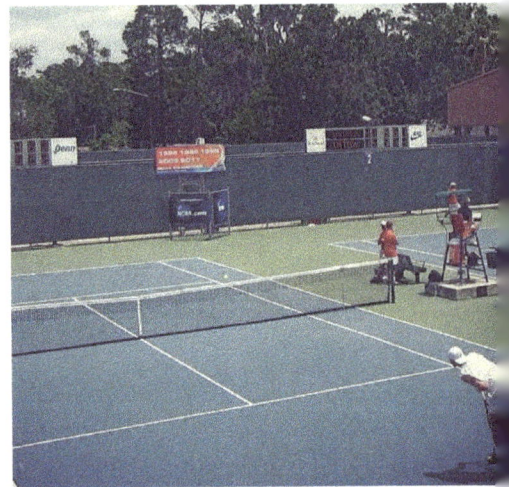

Serving to my opponent at the NCAA's my senior year at Harvard. I have used my background as a tennis player to build the lean body.

If you don't have a background in competitive sports, not to worry—you can still build the lean, athletic body. The strategies in this book, along with the Lean Body Fitness Program in Part IV, will enable you to reach the best shape of your life. Once you have built a strong base of fitness through your lean body workouts, you can then pick up a sport recreationally so as to further develop your functional, enduring physique—not to mention provide you with a change-up every now and again in your training.

Identify Your Optimal Workout

While I outline an all-encompassing approach for getting lean in the pages to come, the path for each individual will be unique. You must tailor the strategies I present to your own body and background to reap the maximum result.

Match your workouts to the physical base you currently have, as well as your sports upbringing. Depending upon your skills, your strengths, and your interests, you will need to make the appropriate adjustments.

Take my own path towards the lean body as an example. I am a tennis player, so before I start my day, I wake up early and complete an intense tennis workout for about an hour and a half. If I can't find somebody to hit with, I'll head to the courts anyway and do footwork, sprints, bodyweight exercises, and finish by hitting serves. Tennis is a great sport because it builds strength, agility, explosive power, and cardiovascular endurance, and whenever I finish my tennis workout I'm completely drained. My background as an athlete has enabled me to build a strong base of aerobic endurance and strength through all of the on-court and off-court training I've done throughout the years. I am now able to use this foundation to train at a high intensity and can complete a draining, full-body workout within a relatively short period of time. That is the ultimate goal for you. Whatever background you have, you must use it to assist you in your current training regimen. If you were a basketball player, for example, use the old routines (sprints, strength, agility) that you used to follow to supplement your lean body program. If you practice yoga, your strength and flexbility will allow you to stay injury free while completing your lean body transformation, so continue your practice on the side.

Tailor your workout plan according to your foundation, and use your background to supplement the program I provide you.

If you don't have a sports background, your first step should be building the base for an athletic body—and we will cover these strategies in the chapters to come. The first step will be to start running every morning for 15-20 minutes before breakfast. After a few months, you can then increase your runs to 25-30 minutes, supplementing them with the lean body strength routines that are laid out in Part IV of the book.

If you already have a good physical base (from time spent in the gym or running outdoors) but haven't been an athlete, use your knowledge and well-conditioned body to take up a sport as a supplement to this program. Enroll in a tennis clinic. Find a soccer game. Play some squash or raquetball. Head to the beach this summer for volleyball. Jump on the field for ultimate frisbee. Leaning down through sports is much more enjoyable than simply following a set workout program, although sticking to the basics will always be necessary.

Keep It Simple

Building the lean body is about executing effective, logical strategies on a consistent basis, and then reaping the results.

Use your body in the way it was intended to be used. Feed your body the food it was designed to process. Get proper rest when your body needs it.

Leaning down is incredibly simple once you know what to do. And it's a very logical process too. Losing weight isn't as complicated as these exercise and diet companies want you to think. Why would they want to make it seem easy? They're making billions from the notion that losing weight is hard and that you need extensive help, hand-holding, and (their) products to do it.

A friend came to me recently because he wanted to lose fifteen pounds. The first piece of advice I gave him was to run 15 minutes before breakfast, and 15 minutes before dinner. "Running is catabolic and I need to focus on building muscle mass so that I'm burning more fat at rest," my friend responded. "I need to go to the gym to do strength and manage macros for body type. I'm an endomorph so I need to keep carbs lower than an ectomorph would."

My friend had been brainwahsed by the nonsense and complications that are so prevalent in modern fitness propaganda. I needed over an hour to convince him to try out the running program. He eventually gave in and has since lost 20 pounds.

Building the lean body involves running and sweating. It requires following through with strenuous workouts and burning off stored fuel in your system. Unfortunately, if you're truly determined to get lean, you can't bank on "burning fat at rest." You need to burn the fat by moving your body.

Sure, leaning down will require discipline and hard work, but once you start building momentum you'll see that you aren't far off. Committing and doing the right things day in and day out will get you there.

Get Down and Dirty

There's no way around it, getting lean means you're going to have to get "down and dirty"—in a workout, a sports match, a grocery shopping, or the preparation of a meal. You need to be willing to invest yourself wholeheartedly in your lean body pursuits, to the point that you forgo any semblance of "keeping it together" or looking good in the act.

During times when I'm completing my workout in the gym and not training outdoors (more to come on why you should move your workout outside whenever possible), I see many gym-goers completing their workouts without breaking a sweat. They comfortably move from one weight machine to the next, or worse, spend their entire time on the elliptical machine. This book won't mislead you by telling you that this is the way to lean down, because it isn't. Sweating as much as you can during your workout should be the goal. If you're drenched by the time you head to the locker room, you've taken a step in the right direction.

You must push yourself in your workouts to the point at which you're fully soaked, covered in dirt, clothes raggedy, and looking the worst you have ever looked. When you walk away from a workout, there's only one thing you should be thinking about: getting into the shower and putting on some dry clothes.

When it comes to your workout attire, the older and more yellowed the clothing, the better—so forget the designer Dri-Fits and LuluLemons (once you attain the lean body, feel free to treat yourself to some nice workout outfits—but until then, a cotton shirt with some holes will be sufficient). One summer during college, I remember playing in a tennis "pro-am" (an event that mixes high level "professional" players—college guys, in this case—with less advanced club members) at a fancy country club before the start of the season. We were forced to wear tennis "whites" (all white clothing) during the exhibition, but my "whites" were actually yellow from all of the times I had sweated in them.

One of the country club members—wearing sparkling clean attire—pointed this out to me during the match. I wasn't embarrassed though. I was proud. The yellowish hue was the proof that I had gotten down and dirty in my training that summer—training that had certainly gotten me leaner, stronger, and ready to perform at my peak for the upcoming season.

Luxury workout environments like upscale gyms that offer towels and cold water at every wall post, along with state-of-the-art air-conditioning systems pumping out sub-zero air, will prevent you from getting lean. Counter the effects of the cold temperature in gyms by working out in a sweatshirt and sweatpants, or if you're able to, find an outdoor field, tennis court, beach, trail, or running track where you can run and complete a series of bodyweight exercises in the heat.

I've learned over the years that the "get down and dirty" mentality can work wonders when you apply it to your life at large, too. If you're studying for an exam, spend hours in the library preparing until your body reeks of the old, mildewed books that surround you. If you're writing a book, don't walk away from the computer until you've finished one or two chapters beyond what you thought was possible that day. If you're preparing a meal for some guests, make sure by the time they arrive, your face and clothes are covered with the raw ingredients you're working with (alright, that's a bit extreme—but you get the idea!). Investing a full, concentrated effort is the only way to accomplish your goals—both in fitness and in life.

Use the Summer to Jump Start Your Lean Body Program

If you happened to pick this book up during the summer, you're in luck.

The summer is a great time to jump start your fitness program because you can exercise outdoors and use the summer heat as a "supplement" to help lean you down. The summer weather promotes sweating, playing sports, and eating an endless variety of healthy fruits and vegetables (nutrition to be addressed in Part II), all of which will contribute to you building a lean, functional physique.

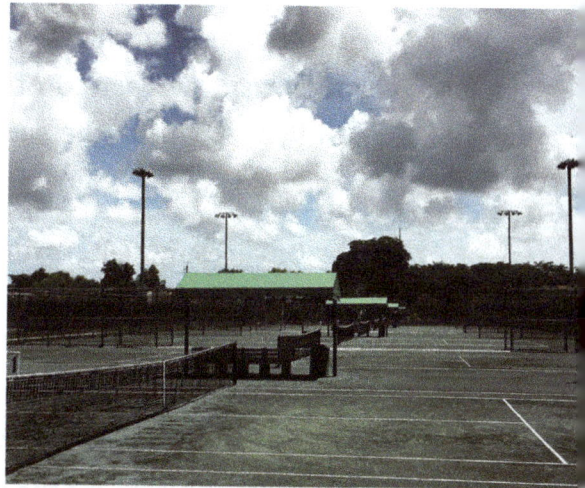

The courts on a sweltering summer day in Florida. Bring your workouts to the outdoors during the summer months to jump-start your lean body progress.

Exercising in the hot weather will increase the physical load on the body by making you work harder, which will up your cardiovascular endurance and overall physical resistance. Working out in the heat, due to the additional effort required, will allow you to achieve a greater volume of work in a shorter period of time.

During my time as a college athlete in the Northeast, I would always try to make it down to the hot and humid weather of Florida to train whenever possible. Returning to school after a trip down south would make me feel like a Superman on the court. I would be moving faster and lighter, and I would never lose my breath.

Training in hot and humid weather and then returning to a colder, less-humid environment is in many ways like taking steroids—only the healthy version. Because the physical volume of work is compressed into a shorter period of time in hot conditions, one hour of practice in heat might be the same as two or three hours in more temperate conditions.

During summer, it's hot everywhere so you don't need to worry about where you are. Just be sure you're using the heat to your advantage by training outside and shedding the excess weight. If it's wintertime, you should aim to simulate the heat of summer by wearing sweatpants and a sweatshirt whenever you work out. By the time June rolls around, you'll be ready to get the most out of your workouts because you'll have become accustomed to training with your body heat elevated.

CHAPTER 2
THE RUN

Rationalizing the Run

To get lean, you need to run. And to get yourself to run, you need to rationalize it.

"Rationalizing the run" means accepting that running is an instrumental and indispensable component of your physical progress. Without the run, you can never build the lean body and master your physicality. People's inability—or refusal—to rationalize the run has led to billions of dollars in revenue for the fitness and health industries, which have presented countless alternatives and quick-fix gimmicks. At the crux of it, if people were out there running and sweating, there wouldn't be such a tremendous demand for exotic diets, complicated exercise programs, and weight loss and fitness fads.

As you know by now, the book you're holding is *not* a quick fix-gimmick or a fleeting attempt at reform. It is a long-term approach that achieves lasting results—results that only come through hard work, discipline, and a logical plan.

You should be running at least four days per week. View it as your breakfast—as a staple component of your daily regimen. Running is the only way you can shed fat and build functional and toned muscles, in addition to speeding up your metabolism, improving your digestion, obtaining a better appetite gauge, and achieving significant cardiovascular endurance.

Whenever I'm in the gym, I often notice people following through with extremely complicated training routines that require the use of all kinds of awkward looking contraptions, even though the best exercise they could do for themselves is to run. One particular instance sticks out in my mind: a young woman going through a routine of push-up "burpees" interspersed with a unique variation of lunges that involved the use of a device resembling a canoe paddle. She had extra weight on her frame and she was struggling to complete these complicated, advanced moves. (As a side note, before I adopted my current program, I too was heavy—20 pounds heavier to be exact—and whenever I tried to do burpees and the like, I struggled. But now that I've achieved a lean frame *through running*, these exercises are a piece of cake.) I interrupted the young woman to explain my own experience.

"Yes, but I just got here after an incredibly long day and I'm too tired," she confided.

This response didn't make much sense, especially given how much she was struggling to complete her routine. But some minutes later she came over to me and voiced the truth: "I hate running!"

The reality is that most people *do* hate running. I used to hate it too. But then I rationalized it. I convinced myself that it was necessary for my progress. This woman—along with many others I often see suffering in the gym at the hands of complicated exercise routines—was trying to overcome her distaste for the run by following through with some other regimen—a regimen that wasn't going to get her the body she wanted. Even more, she was likely harming her joints and tendons in the process because increased weight on the body—especially in advanced body weight exercises and jumps—bears a tremendous burden on these joints and tendons.

Buy a good pair of running sneakers if you don't already have them—and get to it. Understand that running is essential to building a lean, toned, and athletic body. (Note: If running is too hard for you at the outset, work to build up your endurance by using the stationary, *upright* bike and then transition to running once you're stronger. Avoid ellipticals, stair masters, and reclining bikes if you can.)

How to Manage Your Morning Run

Running in the mornings is the first step to getting lean. You must learn how to properly prepare and manage your morning run so that you get the most out of it.

There is a quote I recently saw on Instagram: "I love sleep because it's like a time machine to breakfast." I'm sure we can all relate to this. I know I can. But falling asleep hungry—contrary to what you might otherwise have believed—is *not* the path towards the lean body.

This whole diet fad of restricting food in the evening—and instead eating a large breakfast—is not the best approach. In fact, if you ask many professional athletes (Novak Djokovic for one), they will tell you that they actually don't eat a large breakfast. Rather, these athletes eat normal (if not larger) sized portions at night, fall asleep soundly, and then wake up the next day to burn the calories off from the night before. They're using the stored energy from dinner to fuel their workout the next morning, and this is why they only need a small breakfast portion.

I was brought up—like the rest of America—on the notion that a big breakfast is the best way to start your day. But I've learned and experienced firsthand why eating a small breakfast is actually better: you're lighter, you're not eating when you aren't hungry (appetite isn't usually strong when you wake up in the morning), and you don't have to micromanage your meals during the day to avoid eating a large portion at night.

Managing how much to eat in the evening when you're concerned about your intake is difficult and fragile. You want to eat enough to fall asleep free of pressing hunger, but you also don't want to eat too much. Finding this balance every single day is difficult, if not impossible.

Instead of dealing with the hassle, eat a normal dinner, fall asleep soundly, and then run the next morning. You can even eat two or three *bites* of oatmeal with nuts and dried fruit (raisins, dates, and figs are the best) before your run if you feel you need it.

When I was playing tennis on the professional tennis circuit after college, I noticed that the top-ranked players (mostly European) wouldn't eat very much in the mornings before their matches. At that time, I still was on the "American big breakfast program," and so I couldn't understand how these players could possibly perform eating such a little breakfast. But then I realized: this is *why* they were performing so well. Their bodies had become accustomed to storing the fuel from the prior night's meal and—without a big breakfast weighing them down—they were light and quick on the court come the time of their morning or midday match. One highly-ranked player from France told me that in preparation for his 1pm match, he had only eaten four slices of toast with jam around 9am—and he also warmed up before the match for a full hour too!

I knew I had to change my own habits. Within a couple years (it definitely took time before my body accommodated), I was able to complete a morning match or follow through with a long practice on only few bites of breakfast food. This demonstrates that the body can effectively use the previous night's meal to complete an extended workout in the morning or midday.

If you have to be at work or class by 9 o'clock, this is how your eating schedule and run should work:

Night before: normal meal where you eat to satiety and then fall asleep soundly. Also, prepare your breakfast the night before and pack it up to take with you the next day.

Morning: wake up at 7 o'clock and start your run right away (take a couple bites of oatmeal before if you want). Your run should last 20-30 minutes, and you should stretch for 10 minutes after. Shower, change, and head out the door with your breakfast in hand. With blood still circulating throughout your body (and out of your stomach) from the run, you won't be hungry immediately after.

By the time you get to work or class, hunger should have come on forcefully. Eat your food then and there, as you work or as you listen to the lecture. You won't be fired or kicked out of a class for eating—and if you are, you need to find a new job or professor.

Now you've got your run in. You've burned off the calories from the prior night's dinner. And you're eating a healthy meal to replenish yourself. With strong hunger pressing on by the time you eat in the late morning, you'll have a better gauge on how much to eat and you'll enjoy your food even more.

Maintain a High Intensity

When you hit the field, track, or treadmill (preference of running surface is in that order), you want to make sure you're pushing hard. By the time you're done, you should have nothing left in the tank.

During my senior year at Harvard, in preparation for the pro tennis circuit, I worked to build up my aerobic endurance with a professional runner— Tim Bayley—who was living in Boston

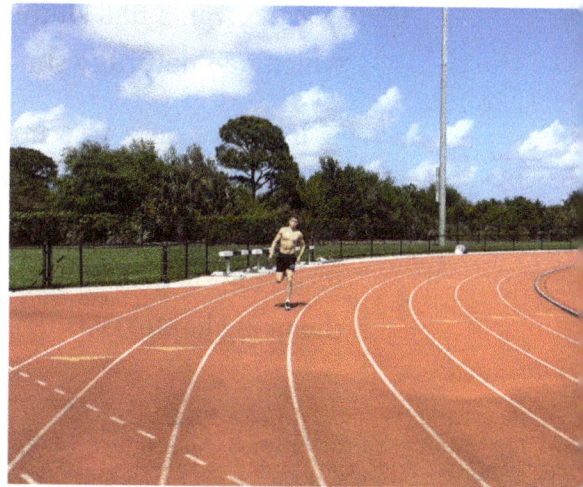

To maintain a high intensity throughout your run, you must cognitively up your pace at distinct markers. If you're running on the track, try to run faster each time you hit the "curve."

at the time. We worked out three times a week early in the morning before classes, and it was then that I began to understand the intricacies involved in maintaining a highly intense run.

When you're running long distances, it's a natural tendency to fade out as the run progresses. The body gets tired and the pace slows. Tim taught me that you need to cognitively up your pace at distinct markers throughout. At the time, I was training on a 200-meter indoor track, and when I would do longer sets of multiple laps, I would make a cognitive effort to up my pace every hundred meters (every half lap). As soon as I hit the "curve" (the semi-circle where the track laps around), I could hear Tim yelling from a distance, "Alright, buddy—now push it!" While I made an extra effort to push harder when he yelled, the end result was neutral: I had simply brought myself back up to the original pace, which had naturally started to lag.

If you're on a treadmill, you don't need a cognitive effort because the machine keeps pace for you. But you want to avoid the treadmill if you can and seek out soft surfaces outside, such as grass and terrain. A forgiving surface will preserve the joints and tendons (more on this in the next chapter).

Finish Strong

It's not only crucial to push yourself during the run, but it's equally important to do so at the end. Leaning down entails finishing your run strong because the last few minutes are what make or break a workout.

Let's assume you're completing a 30-minute run on the treadmill. If you're running at an intense pace for your fitness level (you might need some time to figure out your ideal pace, but the general rule is that you should feel slightly uncomfortable throughout your run, but still have enough energy to keep pushing), you should start to feel the fatigue settling in around the 20 or 25-minute marker.

In my own runs on the treadmill, when I reach 25 minutes, I'm definitely feeling it. Any previously-cooled air has dissipated (I work out in my building gym and am able to turn off the AC completely when nobody's around), and my sweatshirt and sweatpants are keeping my body heat elevated even further. My body surely wouldn't object to a swift punch of the emergency-stop button then and there. But those last five minutes are what boost endurance and burn fat, so stopping isn't an option.

In order to push through, I resolve that I won't look at the clock. Instead, I focus straight ahead and count slowly down from sixty to zero in my head, so slowly that each number probably lasts three or four seconds and five or six strides (sometimes I even cover the treadmill clock with my towel to make certain I don't see the time). By the time

I'm done with the countdown and finally glance at the clock, I'm usually somewhere north of 29 minutes, and tackling those last few seconds is manageable.

It's important that you don't start this 60-second countdown until you're suffering unbearably. You should run normally until your body feels like it can't go any longer, and only at that moment do you implement this technique.

Another strategy for pushing through at the end of a run is to listen to a single song on your iPod—from start to finish—without looking at the clock. Knowing that a single song will last three or four minutes, you can detach yourself from the time by thinking to yourself: "Just get through this one song and you're done."

The reason these strategies work is because a three or four minute window is manageable to push through, especially when you have a clear idea in your mind when this window will end. By distracting your mind from the time and mentally immersing yourself in the countdown or the song, you remove your thoughts from the pain. You're making a pact with yourself to endure the discomfort for this finite period of time while the distraction lasts. You'll notice that the minutes blur together and don't hurt as much.

Control Your Appetite Through Running

The easiest way to control your hunger is by circulating the blood out of the stomach through exercise. Starving yourself is not a long term solution to weight loss as you will learn in Part II—instead you should consume regular meals and dampen your hunger by going for a short run before these meals.

Let's say you eat a hearty lunch around 1 o'clock. The clock strikes six and you can feel your stomach beginning to growl. Instead of taking in the meal at the first onset of hunger, go for a 20-minute run instead. Getting the heart rate up through cardiovascular-based exercise will right away move the blood out of the stomach and into the muscles and extremities. You will find that your appetite will disappear after a couple of minutes into the run, and likely a new wave of energy will come over you. One relevant point here: Going into an exercise session (especially a run) with a little bit of hunger is ideal.

What's great about going for a run before a meal is that you're not only burning off calories from your prior intake, but you're also extending the lifespan of how long those calories last you—which more generally will enable you to eat less throughout the day (your lunch and dinner will be your main meals, breakfast will be light, and you will be snacking more rarely).

Once you get back from the run, you'll notice that you won't be hungry right away. It will take some time for the blood to re-congregate in the stomach and in turn, for the appetite to re-emerge. Even more, incorporating exercise before eating will also give you a better gauge on your appetite, and you will likely eat less as a result.

Start controlling your appetite by circulating the blood out of the stomach and into the muscles and extremities before meals. Get a good stretch, jump in the shower, and then enjoy your food. By the time you get to your first bite you'll be experiencing a stronger, more pressing hunger—and the food will taste even better.

Start incorporating the run into your everyday routine. Like it or not, it's going to be a requirement for building the lean body.

CHAPTER 3
STAY HEALTHY

Injury is Not a Granted Part of Life

There is a prevalent misperception that growing older necessarily involves injury, surgeries, and doctor's visits. Yet if you build an enduring physique in your younger years—working to build up the body properly through disciplined workouts, rigorous stretching, and a proper diet—there is no reason that you should face injury later on. *The Lean Body Manual* is an approach that prioritizes health above all else—you want to be working out your body now and for many years into the future.

One day at the gym I began speaking with a gentleman in in his mid-fifties. He was doing a light workout on the stationary bike and explained that he recently had arthroscopic surgery. For the time being, he was only able to do a light pedal free of resistance.

"How did you hurt yourself?" I asked.

"I didn't hurt myself, I just had to get my knees cleaned out a bit," he replied. "That's what happens when you get older."

The concept that old age (or even middle age, in the gentleman's case) is guaranteed to be intertwined with physical ailments is simply *not* correct. If you're working out in the right way and caring for your body, there should never come a time when you "just [have] to get [your] knees cleaned out." If you build up the body properly, which includes both the muscles *and the tendons and joints* (it's much more difficult to build up the tendons and joints and we'll discuss why shortly), there is no reason that you should have physical problems as you age.

Also, "building up the body" doesn't just relate to exercise. Even more important is a consistent, drawn-out stretching routine that you complete every day (I provide you with a full stretching program in Part IV). This will work to keep your body loose and limber.

Take the ATP Champions Tour—a tennis circuit that includes many of the retired tennis greats—as an example that old age doesn't have to come intertwined with physical ailments. In order to qualify for the Champions Tour you need to have been a world-ranked #1 singles player, a Grand Slam singles finalist, or a singles player on a champion Davis Cup Team.

Many of the retired players that compete on the Champions Tour are in their fifties (and even older!), just like the gentleman in the gym that day. The difference is that these guys have been working out hard and stretching their physical limits *throughout their entire lives.* Even with all those decades of moving their bodies around a tennis court, these players don't have much (if any) visible wear and tear. They're still healthy and they're still playing. Not just playing but *competing*!

Guillermo Vilas is 62. Bjorn Borg is 58. John McEnroe is 55. And these are just a few. I can say with certainty that none of these guys are getting their knees cleaned out. Why? Because as world-class athletes, they have built up their bodies properly, in a manner that will provide them with health and resilience for the long haul.

Building the lean body isn't just about looking good—it's about instilling the proper routines so that you can stay healthy throughout your life. If you're armed with the right knowledge, you can avoid heading down the path of doctors and surgeries.

Work Out on a Soft Surface

Building the lean body involves working every day to preserve your body so you stay injury-free. No matter how hard you're working out, you always need to make sure that your routine is promoting your long-term health—that way, you can stay lean and fit for many years to come. You should never be missing a workout due to injury.

As you know by now, running is a staple workout of the *The Lean Body Manual.* To preserve your body, your runs should be done on a soft surface when possible—such as a dirt trail or a grass field. While synthetic tracks at colleges and high schools are certainly better than concrete, dirt and grass are

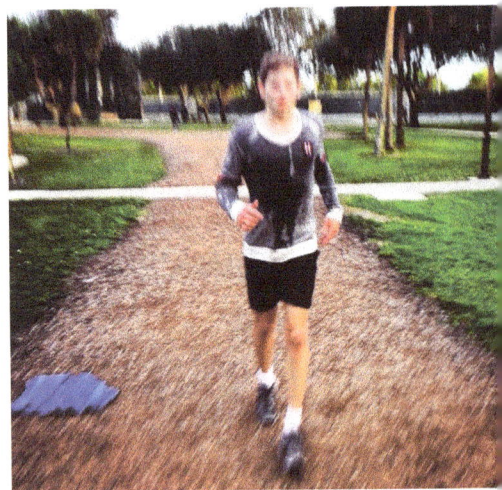

Running on one of the many wood-chip trails in Florida. Seek out a soft surface for your running training whenever possible.

the ideal options. Also, if you have a choice between natural grass and synthetic turf, choose the natural terrain.

Running on a soft surface will be more forgiving on the body and dampen the wear and tear from the ground up, which will enable you to preserve health in your tendons and joints.

In America, most people run on pavement—be it a walking path or road. Even marathon races take place on concrete roads. Without an outsider's perspective, you wouldn't think there was anything wrong with this practice—but it's a plain fact that running on concrete is one of the worst things you can do to your body. As a teenager, I had the good fortune of working with an experienced Hungarian tennis coach—Nandor—who had coached many touring professionals alongside captaining the Fed Cup team for his country. It was Nandor who taught me the benefits of training on a soft surface, and many years later I've realized what priceless advice this was.

If you're a tennis player, you should be playing on a clay court (as opposed to a hard one) whenever possible. This is one reason Florida is such a great place to live, because there are many public clay-court facilities. In contrast, California—another warm-weather tennis destination—only offers hard courts because of the dry climate (the maintenance of a clay court requires consistent watering, which would be too expensive on the West Coast). Recently, I had the opportunity to hit with a famous Hollywood producer in his forties, who was in Boca Raton for the holidays. He is an avid tennis player and told me that he joined the Beverly Hills Tennis Club, paying over $30,000 per year, specifically so he could use the two clay courts there (which are probably the only ones offered in that region). The price was worth it to him because it has made the difference in his ability to stay healthy and keep playing regularly. While the majority can't shell out that type of cash for tennis courts, you can make the conscious choice to play on a clay court if the option is available. Your body will surely thank you.

Pavement is a surface that was meant for cars, never for the human body. The practice of running on concrete has generated billions of dollars for the healthcare sector in the form of hip and knee replacements, ACL tears, achilles tendon ruptures, and other injuries.

In addition to seeking out a soft surface for your workouts, you must pursue an exercise routine that jibes with your current physical condition. For example, if you have excess weight on your frame, it isn't advisable to go running or play tennis right away. Putting a great deal of weight on the joints of the legs (knees, hips, and ankles) will inflict unnecessary wear and tear. Work to burn off the extra weight first through modified nutrition and non-impact exercise such as the stationary bike and swimming. Once you're lighter, find a grass field and take your fitness to the next level through running.

A Proper Warm-Up

A proper warm-up is an integral component of building the lean body. Warming up your body thoroughly before each of your workouts will allow you to stay injury-free so you can work out consistently for the long-haul.

A "proper warm-up" is much more than a two minute jog, a few arm circles, or a quickie hamstring bend. Your warm-up routine should be precise and well thought-out, and should last *at least 10 minutes*. Consider your body to be a tool that needs to be used with precision. Before undertaking any form of exercise, you should understand what your body's needs are so that you won't get hurt. You must be fully confident that at the end of your training session you will walk away healthy.

Use these five tips to complete a proper warm-up: (1) Always run for 5-10 minutes before any workout. (2) Stretch out each of the major muscle groups of the legs (hamstrings, groin, calves, glutes, and quadriceps). (3) Spend two minutes warming up the upper body through arm swings and arm crosses. (4) Wear long sleeve pants and a long sleeve shirt during the warm-up so that your body heat elevates quickly. (5) Do not start any rigorous workout until you have started to perspire. (The full, Lean Body Warm-Up routine is outlined in detail in Part IV.)

In addition to a proper warm-up before exercise, you must work to keep the body warm *during* the workout too. The optimal scenario for this is exercising outdoors during the summer, with the warm sun beating down on you. During the colder months, you should be wearing multiple layers. If you're forced to work out in an air-conditioned gym, make sure to wear appropriate clothing so that the chill doesn't affect you. Cold joints, muscles, and tendons during a workout will pose an injury risk and compromise your long-term health.

Build Up Your Tendons and Ligaments

Strengthening the muscles of the body is the easiest part in your lean body transformation—it's building up the tendons and ligaments of the joints that takes the most time.

The tendons and ligaments require *at least six months* of proper, disciplined workouts before they begin to undergo a transformation. Strengthening these areas is the most important because doing so will allow you to stay healthy over the long-run.

You often see photos in fitness magazines of people who have undergone one or two-month-long workout routines, with the "before and after" shots showing impressive changes. While these people may have doubled the size of their muscles (which itself is unnatural for such a short time period), they've certainly failed to build up the connecting ligaments and tendons to properly support them.

The result? Injury.

Don't be fooled by the allure of a quick body transformation—not only is it dangerous, but it won't last. You want to work consistently over an extended stretch of time so that your body can accommodate and adjust in the right way—one where you stay injury-free for the long haul.

The best way to strengthen the ligaments and tendons alongside your muscles is to start working out with your own body weight. Your workouts—in addition to your daily runs—should involve the strength routines that are laid out in Part IV, which incorporate many bodyweight exercises so you can build yourself up in a sustainable, lasting manner. Working out the body *with the body* will enable you to strengthen the organism in its entirety, instead of simply isolating specific muscle groups on a weight machine.

Invest in the Proper Athletic Footwear

One major component to staying healthy is making sure you have the proper athletic footwear.

Your physical health works its way from the ground up. In the same way you want to work out on a soft surface, you also want to make sure your sneakers are providing proper support and cushioning. Without proper sneakers, the rest of your body—lower back, knees, ankles, and hips—will suffer.

Buying sneakers should be calculated and well thought-out. You should go to a reputable store where the salespeople are knowledgeable about what it is you're looking for. If you're buying running sneakers, go to a running store, or if it's tennis shoes, head to a shop that specializes in tennis. Never order sneakers online without trying them on beforehand.

Let's take an example where you're buying *running* sneakers specifically, but the protocol would apply to all types of athletic shoes. When you arrive at the running store, find a knowledgeable employee who's been working in the store for several years. Have him look at your foot and determine whether it's flat or narrow. Let him measure your foot size (even if you already know it) to determine a precise fit. In one instance, a friend of mine in his thirties had been wearing a size 10 running shoe his whole life, only to find out later on from a knowleddable salesperson that he is actually size 11.5!

It's possible for somebody to make a mistake like this because the ideal fit differs for different kinds of shoes. For example, you should wear a half size larger in running sneakers than tennis sneakers. While running you need additional space in front of the toes, whereas on the tennis court a snugger fit is ideal. Dealing with a shoe vendor that specializes in a particular sport will give you the best chance of finding an optimal sneaker and fit.

Do some research online before heading into the store. Having an idea of the various brands (even if minimal) will provide you with the ability to ask the salesman questions. In certain cases, stores have incentives to sell a particular brand of sneaker, and arming yourself with all possible information is best.

Once you've identified a shoe that fits well, you can save money by purchasing older colors of the same model online (*make sure it's the same model, just in a different color* because if the model itself is older, the fit might be different). Maybe it won't look as cool, but you will be getting down and dirty in your workouts anyway so it doesn't much matter.

CHAPTER 4
RECOVERY

Active Rest

Resting the body properly is just as important as working out hard. In order to get lean, you must listen to your body to determine when it needs to rest because taking off at the right times will prevent you from getting hurt. You also need to understand *how* to properly rest.

Let's suppose you work out all week and take off Saturday and Sunday. In addition to sleeping in and lazing around, you should aim to actively assist your body in the recovery process—in turn preparing yourself for next week's training.

Active rest means tending to the body so that the joints and muscles recover fully during your time off.

The first component of active rest is stretching. On your days off, you want to take a ten minute jog to warm up the body, and then stretch out for at least 20 minutes. This will loosen the body by removing any accumulated tightness from the week. If you cut short some of your stretching sessions during that week's workouts, this is your time to make up for it.

Another component to active rest is massage, which we will address in more detail to come. If you're training hard, you need to get a massage once every two weeks—there's simply no way around it.

In my own experience, when weeks went by without getting a

massage, injury almost always resulted. One example sticks out in my mind: I played a string of professional tennis tournaments in the Midwest. By the fifth tournament (with four weeks of traveling and twelve matches behind me), my upper back muscles and shoulders had accumulated significant tension. Sure enough, during my warm-up the day of the event, I pulled a muscle and was forced to withdraw (this is one reason good tennis coaches will always recommend that you play no more than three tournaments in a row before taking a rest block).

Make sure you go for a swim on your off days (unless your sport *is* swimming!). Swimming assists the body in recovery by loosening the muscles and relieving tension—especially in the back and shoulders (implement the crawl and breast strokes). Simply floating in water will also work wonders for restoring any minor nicks in the body. Whenever I go into the pool—or, even better, the ocean—I feel the positive effect right away.

Lastly, make sure to fuel the body with healthy, nutritious food on your off days. Active rest also means providing the body with the necessary nutrition (covered fully in Part II) so that when the training week starts up again, you're fueled with energy and ready to exert yourself.

Stretching

Stretching is a centerpiece of The Lean Body Fitness Program and it should be regarded with equal importance to your daily run. Stretching improves muscle function, it prevents injury, and it contributes to your Feel Good State (more on the Feel Good State to come). Without a flexible and agile body, you will remain incapable of maximizing your physical potential.

Strangely—even with the weight loss, fitness, and diet craze of today—nobody seems to be advocating the importance of stretching. Stretching is the one piece of the puzzle that has gone overlooked.

After each workout you should be stretching for *at least 15 minutes*. While you should follow a routine of dynamic stretching (short 2-3 second stretches interspersed with movement) before your workout, the bulk of your stretching should be done *after* your training because this is when the muscles will be fully warm. You will also be able to feel your body better after you've worked out, and can therefore target the specific areas

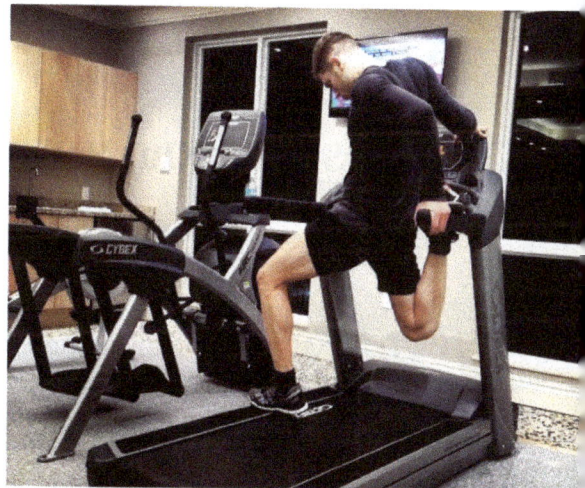

The bulk of your stretching should be done after your workout. Make sure you stretch your body out for at least 15 minutes.

of your body that feel particularly tight. Whenever I spend time at the gym or on the tennis court, I rarely see a person actually taking his or her stretching seriously. Stretching shouldn't be an afterthought—it should be an integral component of your routine.

My own stretching routine and the flexibility it provides has enabled me to stay healthy for the last ten years. I make sure to never walk off the court or field without stretching out each muscle group thoroughly. As a result, I have been able to transform my body into that of a high level athlete without any injuries.

My full stretching routine—including the dynamic stretching for your warm-up—is included in Part IV. Study it and learn it inside out. This is your gateway to the lean body.

Stretch Out Your Back

In all of the years I've frequented gyms, tracks, and tennis courts, I've never seen somebody spend the time to stretch out his or her back—surprising given how common back injuries are. Back injuries are known to afflict tennis players especially, and are a scourge among the middle-aged and elderly.

As a fifteen year-old, I had the opportunity to practice with Tarik Benhabiles, the former coach of Andy Roddick, and it was he who showed me the back stretch I now do religiously (and have been doing for the last decade). Tarik, then in his mid-forties, was still stretching out his back every day and he repeatedly stressed it would be the game-changer in my tennis career.

The stretch is simple: Get on the ground with both legs extended out in front of you, and then bring your legs over your head until your toes touch the ground, holding for upwards of ten seconds (part IV includes pictures showing this stretch).

Before I complete this stretch, I usually lean forward to stretch out my hamstrings first. I find that releasing tension in the hamstrings beforehand makes the back stretch more effective (you'll also find that loose hamstrings will relieve tension in the lower back as well).

In the beginning you'll likely feel the stretch in the mid or upper back (and you might have difficulty touching your feet to the ground at first). Keep working at it. Once you've perfected this stretch, your feet should touch the ground and you should be feeling the release primarily in the *lower* back region—which is ideal because it is the lower back in particular that is prone to injury.

As with all components of *The Lean Body Manual*, the key to you securing a loose back is *consistency* in your stretching routine. Do it every day. Times when I've failed to stretch my back for periods longer than a few days, my feet would no longer touch the ground. Moreover, my movement on the tennis court would suffer because added tension in the back increases tension throughout the body.

Securing a Worthwhile Massage

To build the lean body, you will need to get a massage once every two weeks—and selecting a good massage therapist is crucial. You need a therapist who's knowledgeable about the body and who can provide you with a quality service.

How do you select a good massage therapist? Part of it is trial and error, and the other part is getting in touch with your body so that you know good from bad yourself. By working out consistently and taking care of your body through regular stretching and healthy food, you will increase the strength of your proprioception (how you perceive and feel your own body), which will in turn allow you to gauge the quality of your massage.

Ask these three questions to determine if your massage therapist is the right one: (1) Is the pressure of the massage deep enough that you feel slightly uncomfortable throughout the massage? If so, good. (2) Do you feel comfortable communicating with the massage therapist *during the massage* about what he's doing right and what he needs to change? If so, good. (3) When you come out of the room, do you feel like something was missing from the massage? Is there still lingering tightness or does something feel incomplete? If so, this is bad.

Massage is important because it loosens and releases tension within the muscles and it will ensure you don't get injured—and can continue your workout routine day in and day out. It will also revitalize and restore the mind, not just from the effects (and pleasure) of the massage itself, but also from the knowledge that you're doing a great thing for your body and your health.

How do you know if the pressure is enough in the massage? To start with, you should never be comfortable at any point in the massage. The pressure should be such that any slight increase would cause great discomfort. You want manageable discomfort so that you're constantly on the edge. It's difficult to find this balance because sometimes the therapist will work too light, and other times too hard. This is why a constant dialogue with the therapist during the massage is important—it's *you* who needs to communicate when you need more pressure and when you need less.

You're getting a good massage if your nose gets stuffy midway through. Nasal congestion indicates you're experiencing inflammation in the body—a sign the massage is doing the job. Adhere to this rule: If you don't blow your nose at least once during the massage, it was not an effective one.

Get Your Boyfriend or Girlfriend to Massage You

Paying for regular massages can be expensive and the reality is that you don't always need a full-body massage from a professional—especially if you have tightness only in one specific area. When your problem is localized, it's fine if a non-professional steps in—namely, your boyfriend or girlfriend.

Next time you come home from your lean body-building workout, tell your partner to turn off the TV and come into the bedroom. Put on some relaxing music. Light a candle if you feel inclined. Then get out some massage oil and have him or her rub you down where it hurts. Then return the favor.

When your partner massages you, it's important you maintain heightened awareness of what he or she is doing. The last thing you want is to get hurt from too much pressure being exerted on the wrong part of the body.

Getting your boyfriend/girlfriend to massage you is a win-win. Not only will you be working to heal each other, but the sensual experience could very well lead to some other very healthy activity.

Roll Out on a Lacrosse Ball

To loosen up the body fully, you'll need to use a lacrosse ball to "roll out" tight areas that can't be targeted through stretching.

The lacrosse ball is the perfect tool because it's solid and small—and so you can exert extreme pressure on small surface areas of the body. Position yourself on a yoga mat and use the ball while lying down on the floor. Once you have pinpointed an area of tightness, lean into the ball with your body weight, exerting pressure on that specific location. Move the ball around slightly so you can tackle the surrounding area as well.

I implement the lacrosse ball to loosen my hips, glutes, shoulders, and bicep tendons. Roll yourself out after workouts when the blood is circulating and you can feel exactly where you need it.

Take a Bath

In tending to the body outside of workouts, baths are an extremely useful tool. Baths—and being in water more generally—promote muscle-recovery and work to heal lingering aches and pains. The two baths that you should implement are (1) ice baths and (2) Epsom salt baths.

Before arriving at college, I had never heard of or used an ice bath—yet during my time at both Brown and Harvard I would often see other athletes using them in the training room. In travelling to other sports facilities while competing, I noticed nearly every college had one.

Ice baths are useful as a post-workout recovery tool, the logic being that they reduce inflammation and flush out lactic acid from the muscles by constricting blood cells.

I began using ice-baths consistently during my junior year at Harvard, usually two or three times a week after intense practice sessions or long matches. I can attest to their effectiveness first hand. Most of the athletes (including myself) were using the bath for their legs primarily, and I would often find myself sharing the tub with several runners on the track team.

You don't need a college athletic training room for an ice-bath—it's easy to make one at home. Take a 10lb bag of cubes and dump it into the bath tub. Fill it up with some cold water and jump in for *not more than ten minutes.*

In addition to ice baths, you should be taking warm baths with Epsom salt (magnesium sulfate) added. Epsom salt works to soak out toxins from the body, thereby reducing swelling and relaxing muscles.

It's always hard to find time to take a bath, but doing so will contribute immeasurably to your success in building the lean body.

Care for Your Feet

We've already discussed the importance of buying the proper athletic footwear in the last chapter—and it's equally important to wear the right shoes outside of your training. The last thing you want is to suffer an injury from poor-quality or bad-fitting leisure shoes.

Many times I've suffered from foot problems provoked by bad footwear worn *outside* of my training sessions and competitions. I now understand the importance of a good pair of leisure shoes (walking, loafers, or dress) that have sufficient cushioning and fit well.

In one example, I bought a pair of the "Nike Breathe Free" sneakers—a light-weight model that compromises on support. These shoes provoked a sharp pain at the forefoot and cost me several weeks of training. In another example, I purchased a pair of "Gola" sneakers online that resulted in heel problems—again forcing me to stay off the tennis court for some time. In both instances, the pain crept on slowly and I didn't initially realize what was causing it. By the time I did, the damage had already been done.

Sneakers should always be purchased for the fit, not the style. Do your best to look cool, but never sacrifice your foot health for some trendy design.

The lean, athletic body will only come from a consistent workout routine where you're on your feet moving and so foot injuries are nearly impossible to work around.

PART II:
PERFECT YOUR
NUTRITION

CHAPTER 5
OVERCOME THE MODERN FOOD LANDSCAPE

Let's Get 1970s Lean

Over the last few years I've developed a taste for 1970s music—the Bee Gees, the Ramones, and Earth, Wind & Fire. I've downloaded all of their songs and perused many YouTube videos of performances during their heyday. I could not believe how lean these guys looked!

All of these artists—including other popular bands of the era—were rail-thin—no noticeable body fat on them—with waists probably measuring 29 inches. When you compare the way these guys looked in the '70s to the way people look today, it's like examining two different species. Of course, there are still thin people in the world today, but the thin "look" of the '70s bands was different—it was a healthy-looking thin (John Travolta looks the same way in the famous film *Saturday Night Fever*). When you compare how thin people look today, they seem emaciated and malnourished.

The 70s bands would probably come off stage after a four-hour performance and—despite having zero reserves in the form of fat—not even feel hungry (granted, they were most likely doing a few drugs too).

The bands looked different than the people of today because *they were different*. In the '70s, only 12% of the population was obese—compared with over 36% today, a number that's only rising. Humans haven't changed biologically—so what happened?

Like me, all of my friends are in their mid to late twenties now—and it's an unfortunate fact that already the weight has started to pile on. A strange correlation: the more bloated the face and the larger the stomach, the more hair seems to have been lost.

And my friends aren't even living such unhealthy lifestyles! They're eating out at restaurants a couple of times a week, maybe having a few drinks on the weekend. That's standard behavior, yet even so the effects of this moderately unhealthy lifestyle are alarming.

There's something out there that's causing these physical changes—changes that more or less have been accepted by society as a granted facet of the aging process (even for young adults). So what's changed?

The modern food landscape differs greatly from that of previous decades—the stuff's more processed, it has less nutrition, it's more addicting, and it's unhealthier.

I am convinced that the new-age food is the culprit—and my expertise is overcoming the physical effects that it provokes. To be healthy within the modern food landscape, extreme measures have to be undertaken. It's all or nothing when it comes to perfecting your nutrition and fostering real changes for the long haul. And that's because of how addicting this food is. It's simply too powerful. One bad meal will ignite the cravings engine for weeks going forward and obliterate any progress you've made.

Will we ever get back to the physiques of the 1970s? As a society, probably not. But that doesn't mean *you* can't. With some focus, dedication, and determination—along with the lessons to be set forth— you can be the exception. The loner. The only person out there in a vast sea of bloated faces and blossoming bellies with a waistline comparable to the 1970s bands—and looking healthy while doing it, not starving or sickly.

It's time to focus on the important things. To invest your energy into—as the Bee Gees put it—"Stayin' Alive." But in a very literal sense.

Let's get to it. There's no more time to waste.

Eat to Live. Don't Live to Eat.

When it comes to your eating, you need to enjoy your food and take pleasure in your daily meals. Yet there's a fine line between eating because you *need* to and eating because you *want* to. "Wanting" to eat means you're eating because you're experiencing food cravings and "needing" to eat means your body is actually lacking nutrition.

The only way to rid the body of the wanting is to eschew the processed, addictive, and scientifically-engineered foods offered in mainstream food destinations. These foods are like drugs—and it isn't by chance. They're meticulously crafted to produce the "high" you experience and once you're fully consumed by them, there's simply no coming out (unless, of course, you're reading this book).

I saw a telling Facebook post that presented a "relationship status" survey question listing, "Single," "Married," "It's complicated," and "In a relationship," with the final checkbox reading "In line at Chipotle." The final option was ticked. This metaphor of *Chipotle as a romantic path* indicates the unnerving reality of just how addicting and powerful these food options are.

Before I adopted the diet plan that I now follow, I too was invested in the mainstream food culture—Chipotle naturally included. I loved Chipotle and whenever I would go, I felt like I could just plant myself at one of those metallic tables and sit there eating for hours. The combination of the saltiness, sour cream, sauces, and fatty meat would transport me to some other place, just like lab technicians intended it to. This stuff will satisfy any craving you have and then some—maybe even give a purpose to your life (coming back for more). It's too damn good!

When you're eating food that's too damn good, you're going to face food cravings and you're going to be *wanting* to eat. You're going to be *living* to eat.

In the chapters to come, we will work to move your check from the "Chipotle line" to another status. Doesn't matter which other option you select, so long as you're craving romantic release and *not* food-craving release.

The time has come to start eating to live.

The Consequences of the Unhealthy Meal

Eating an unhealthy meal isn't just harmful because the food is bad for you—it's harmful because it sets you up for a cycle of cravings and hunger. When someone caves for pizza and says—"Oh, it's just a couple of slices, it's not going to hurt me"—this person is failing to understand the double-edged sword of an unhealthy meal in the modern food landscape.

Unhealthy mainstream food hits you from two angles, the first being food cravings. The combination of high salt, sugar, and fat ignites the ravenous animal within. You're going to want more of this food and you're going to eat a large portion when you sit down to it—there's simply no way around it. And when the next day rolls around, you're still going to be thinking about it—and you'll mobilize to get more. These foods will fully and mercilessly consume you, in turn leading you to consume them.

The second angle comes from the hunger, which results from your body not receiving the proper (if any) nutrients. Why are you still hungry after

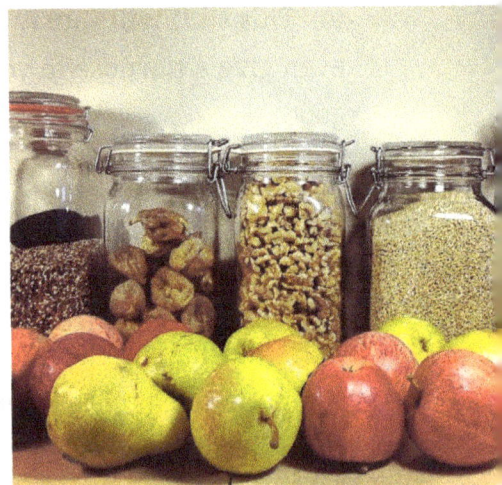

Fresh apples and pears, dried figs, walnuts, and grains. To get lean you will need to move away from mainstream food options and start cooking at home.

three Big Macs? The reason is that your body isn't getting the necessary nutrition, despite your having consumed a few thousand calories. A nutrition-starved body is dangerous because you will constantly be hungry. Your body will be compromised and you will likely suffer from fatigue, random bouts of illness, and a subpar lifestyle overall.

In my own experience, when I eat healthy food after eating unhealthily, I'm usually eating a lot more when I sit down to the healthy food. The reason for this is because my body—conditioned to having the proper nutrition from a healthy diet—is trying to compensate for the lack of nutrition from the prior meal. *And this is just from one meal!*

To do away with cravings and hunger you need to provide the body with proper nutrition. The unhealthy meal needs to be a thing of the past.

Forget the Restaurant

The first step towards mastering your nutrition is to forget the restaurant. To truly lean down, you must cook your meals at home.

Getting into the habit of preparing your own food will work wonders for your physique. It doesn't even matter if you cook relatively "unhealthy" food at the start—simply by avoiding restaurants you will begin seeing immediate changes in how you look and feel.

Whenever I do go out to dinner—which is rare—I usually feel great going into the meal and am looking forward to it (interspersing some restaurant meals into your program will be necessary down the road—to keep yourself sane, if nothing else—but for now, stick to the eat-at-home program). I can always feel the effects of a restaurant meal the morning after, however, almost like a hangover. My fingers and eyelids are swollen from the excess salt. I'm not as energized as I normally am getting up and starting my day. I'm thirsty. I feel heavy in my morning workout.

When you eat restaurant food after having prepared your own meals for a while, your taste buds will explode. You'll likely become immersed in the flavors and seemingly lose track of where you are. You'll be transported to another world and everything around you will become blurred together in a thick haze as you experience the all-consuming flavors. Stepping away from restaurant food for some time and then coming back to it will show you firsthand just how powerful and addicting those offerings are.

Normally when I eat a healthy meal at home, I'm not drinking much water alongside the food. Natural foods are filled with water and they contain very little salt. But whenever I eat out, I often find myself drinking several glasses of water throughout the sit down. Add onto this the fact that salt—which restaurant food has plenty of—retains water in the body. The combination will soon inflate your body with excess fluid, the exact opposite from the lean body that we're aiming for.

Going out to restaurants regularly (or ordering food in) will empty out your wallet quickly. Even with the premium that you pay, the ingredients at restaurants aren't top of the line. The food usually isn't organic. Most of the time the fish isn't wild caught, and the steak isn't "grass fed"—which are the ideal. Certainly the oils they cook with aren't optimal (olive oil is the best). You might as well save your money and buy the best possible ingredients for your home-cooked meals. Then invest your extra cash into a new pair of running sneakers or a tennis racquet, and start getting lean.

Get Rid of Cheese and Wheat

There's little room for debate here: cheese is heavy, it's fattening, it's highly-caloric and it's going to weigh you down. Getting rid of the cheese is the first step in ridding dairy completely from your life, which will be necessary if you want to get lean.

Cheese has become the primary source of fat in the American diet, in large part due to food industry marketing. Cheese was once a delicacy to be enjoyed with guests before a meal, but it has now become a common ingredient that is used in everyday life, often multiple times per day. Unlike whole milk, full-fat cheese doesn't visually appear to be a high fat food. Manufacturers have used cheese's seemingly innocent nature to push it onto consumers—walking around the grocery store you will find cheese being sold in every form imaginable (dips, creams, spreads, sticks, balls, crackers, crisps, chips, etc.)

Getting rid of cheese (and other dairy products) in my own life has had a significant effect in shedding excess weight. Within a couple months of abstaining from cheese I had lost 10 pounds, and it has stayed off ever since.

Similarly, you've got to give up the wheat too—and that includes most breads. The blood sugar high and insulin response that follows the consumption of wheat has provoked the large stomach syndrome (visceral fat accumulation) we see in society today. If you want a flat (lean) stomach, you must replace bread and wheat pastas with other carbohydrates—whole grains and fruit primarily (discussed in more detail to come).

Preparing and storing cooked grains in your fridge at home will be the first step away from wheat. On weekends, you should boil large batches of brown rice, quinoa, steel-cut oats, and buckwheat so that you have these on hand for the week. Grains should be used to complement all of your meals—and eating these grains will prevent hunger throughout the day.

Buy some Pyrex containers so you can bring a batch of grains along with you during the day. If you're forced to eat out with co-workers or friends for lunch, order a salad and mix the grains in.

Healthy Fats

To build the lean body, you need to replace unhealthy fats with healthy ones—swapping out the 20-ounce rib-eye for a piece of wild salmon, for example.

Healthy fat comes from nuts, fish, avocado, and healthy oils (olive oil is my go-to).

When it comes to nuts, you should be eating them whole (not in "butter" form). When you're forced to chew the nuts, you will have a better gauge on how much to eat and won't overdo it. Buy Brazil nuts, almonds, pecans, and walnuts.

Get some fresh, wild fish low in mercury: sardines, cod and flounder are great options. You can throw these into the oven or onto the steamer and they'll cook quickly—usually in less than 10 minutes.

Start eating avocados (I usually eat at least half of an avocado for both lunch and dinner). Add them to salad and grains. If you're eating a piece of wheat-free bread (buy the "Mestemacher" or

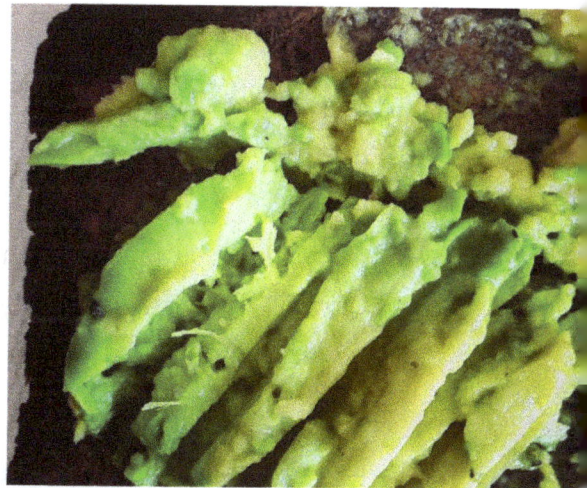

Avocado spread onto a piece of Mestemacher bread. Two key secrets to attaining the lean body: avoid wheat and replace your butter with avocado.

"Dimpflmeier" brands), use a ripened avocado as your "butter."

Start sautéing your vegetables in olive oil. If you don't have the time to cook a fresh batch of grains, you can add pre-cooked grains from the fridge directly into a vegetable sauté for a quick, hot, and delicous meal. (Whenever possible, try to add your pre-cooked grains directly into the dish you're preparing on the stovetop, as opposed to heating them up in the microwave. Microwaves diminish the nutritional quality of your food.)

Eating healthy fats will make your skin look better. Your hair will be healthier. Your nails will be stronger. Your inner workings will be lubricated. Your joints will function optimally.

Eat a Full Meal

There's a saying: "Athletes don't diet and exercise. They eat and train."—and to get lean, you must think like an athlete. You should be working out hard and then supplying the body with proper nutrition afterwards.

The prevalent mainstream approach to thinking about food as "calories"—and then seeking to restrict those calories—isn't the way to go. Cutting calories (unless you're truly overeating) shortchanges the body of the nutrients it needs to function optimally. You'll be hungry every day and your life will be compromised as a result. Your workouts will be lacking because you won't have enough fuel to push hard, and you will suffer mentally because you won't be able to fully concentrate and stay in the moment.

Contrary to typical diet book advice, you should actually eat to satiety—but only eat nutritious and healthy foods. In this way, every "calorie" consumed has value. Each piece of food put inside your body is providing some mineral, ingredient, or vitamin that will help boost your body's functionality.

When you sit down to eat, you should consume a "full meal." A full meal is comprised of whole grains, vegetables, and a piece of fish or meat (50% grains, 30% vegetables, and 20% meat/fish). In order to get lean, you must focus on the *proportion of the portion*. Eating the right proportion of food at each and every sit-down will allow you to eat less in the long-run. You won't overeat, and you'll see with time that you won't need as much food to feel full (and that's the goal: to decrease the daily amount of food you need to sustain yourself).

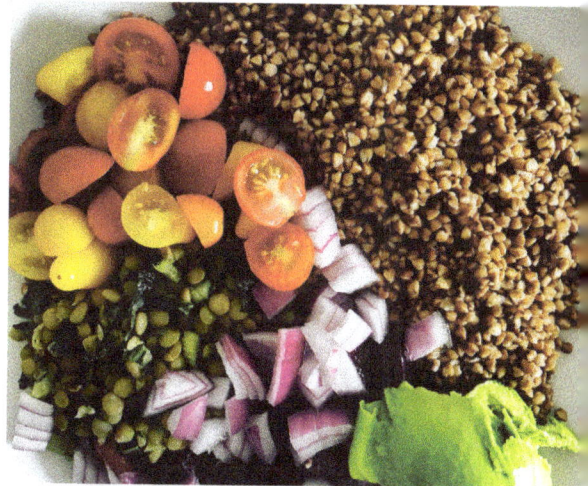

A full vegetarian plate: kasha, chopped cherry tomatoes, red onion, beets, lentils with kale, and avocado.

You can choose to make your plate fully vegetarian by replacing your fish or meat serving with a whole avocado, which will make you feel completely satisfied. Always feel free to add avocado slices to complement a full plate that includes protein (in general, never worry about how much avocado you're eating).

Whole grains (quinoa, brown rice, wild rice, buckwheat, brown rice pasta, and steel-cut oats) and vegetables should be the foundation of your nutritional program—and when you eat fish or meat, the piece shouldn't exceed 6 ounces. With a consistent daily workout regimen, it will be impossible for you to gain weight because you'll be "eating and training"—just like an athlete.

Fad diets, complicated cleanses, and carb-cutting regimes are not the solution. Take the "Paleo" diet as an example—where you don't eat grains but instead fill up on meat, vegetables, and fruit. To avoid hunger on this diet, you'll need to eat huge quantities of food (and meat, in particular)—rendering your body heavy and bulky. Eating a full meal with the correct proportions will allow you combat hunger throughout the day while eating less overall because you'll be satiated, energized, and focused on daily tasks instead of needing to snack every hour.

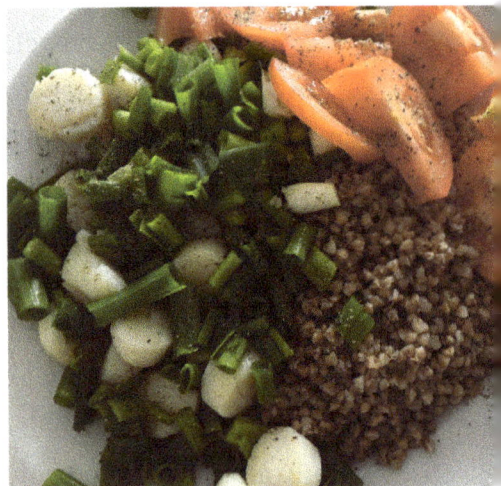

Be sure you eat a full meal every time you sit down. Here is a plate of kasha (buckwheat), steamed scallops, tomato, and chopped scallions. Half an avocado will be added on the side.

What's more is that the meat industry today is horrible. Animals are treated poorly—they're cooped inside small cages, fed antibiotics and other chemical-laden substances, slaughtered inhumanely (often times still conscious and feeling pain), and prevented from ever seeing the light of day. It's difficult to cut out meat entirely from your diet, but you can take the necessary steps to limit your intake. Doing so will help you get lean, avoid the byproducts (antibiotics, etc.) inside meat that then enter your own body, *and* make a statement against the current methods of the industry.

Take Control of Your Bowels

Once you begin to consume the proper foods, not only will you look and feel better, but you'll also benefit from a regular release of the bowels. Relieving the bowels should be a one-time affair done each day first thing in the morning, in which your entire intestine is cleared out for a 24-hour period.

Several bathroom trips during the course of a day are not separate bowel movements. They are a single one spread out over the course of multiple trips. This is the result of a compromised excretory system that's having difficulty processing what you've given it, so it's failed to establish a natural Circadian rhythm.

Processed and unnatural foods, along with dairy and wheat, result in bowels that are hard and intact—and will never facilitate a once-a-day, 3-minute sitting. Take the burden off your digestive track and provide it with the food it was intended to process: natural foods comprised of single ingredients. Giving your body a chance will allow it to work its magic and establish regularity.

Not having to worry about nature calling during the course of your day is reason enough to start making the right food choices. You'll have peace of mind knowing that you won't have to sprint to the water closet in the middle of your big presentation.

The proper nutrition will make you feel better, look younger, and live longer. Many psychologists even believe that mental health stems from the health of the intestine, so you may be able to increase mental acuity and ward off depression as well.

There's no better feeling than living your days with a clear intestine. Establishing regularity should be reason enough to start eating healthy, nutritious food. But on top of that, you'll also be moving yourself closer towards the lean body.

CHAPTER 6
PREPARE YOUR FOOD

Pursue a Sustainable Approach

Cold-pressed juice has become a phenomenon in the last decade. In Florida where I live, new stores sprout up every year. Whenever I return to New York City, my hometown, I notice a new cold-pressed juice shop on every corner. While the logos, pamphlets, and fancy drink names may appeal and seem to offer a solution to the modern weight loss conundrum, the path of juicing will never allow you to master your physicality and get lean. At the end of the day, nobody—doesn't matter who you are—can sustain him or herself on cold-pressed juice alone and go on to live a fully-optimized, cognitively-attuned, hunger-free life.

Consumers are misled by juicing stores and made to believe that it's possible to sustain the body on these juices alone. They remain in the dark about how to manage their nutrition in a healthy, sustainable manner. There's no way around it: to build the lean body, you need to take the time to sit down and consume a full meal. Without the proper sustenance, you will remain incapable of pushing through the lean body-building workouts.

In the pages to come, you will learn a realistic and sustainable strategy for controlling your hunger through the consumption of healthy, nutritious foods—whole grains included. But hey—if you absolutely must have a $12 cup of juice along the way, nobody's going to stop you.

Be Prepared

Getting lean involves being prepared. You need to be on top of things—whether it's preparing for a workout by warming up, or preparing your food for the day to come so you don't end up at the local fast food joint.

It's crucial you have healthy food on hand when hunger strikes because that's when you make bad food choices. Keep your refrigerator stocked. Cook your lunch the night before and bring it with you to work or class. Bring along an apple during your afternoon errands. The minute you become hungry without the proper food accessible is the same minute you will start destroying all the progress you've made up until that point. All it takes is one bad meal to head down the path of food cravings and weight gain.

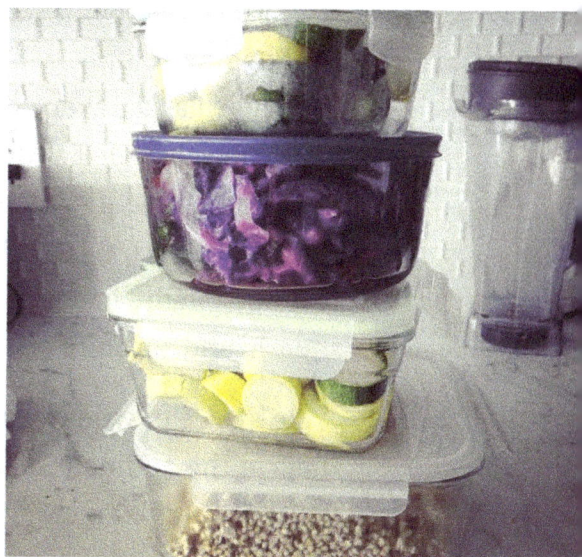

Food preparation is key to leaning down. Kasha and steamed vegetables in several Pyrex containers.

If you're working out hard, you'll get incredibly hungry in a moment. You need to accept this fact and take the necessary steps to have healthy food and snacks with you at all times. Combining proper workouts with the right nutrition is the only way to advance, and so taking your food preparation seriously is a must.

Force Yourself to Eat Healthy

A great way to force yourself to eat healthy is to buy large quantities of healthy food when you go to the market. Having fresh produce, fish, meat, and fruits in the refrigerator will pressure you to consume it because you won't want your food (and money) to go to waste.

Identify a local market with reasonable prices and then head there each week to fill up your kitchen with fruit and vegetables (try to buy organic if possible). The high markups at brand name supermarkets such as Whole Foods and The Fresh Market will empty your pocket quickly, so try to avoid these overpriced stores if you can.

Shopping in bulk will also save you time from having to stop into the supermarket every other day—just be sure to keep track of what you've purchased. Eat the vegetables that go bad quickly first—lettuce, bok choy, and leafy greens (kale, chard, dandelion greens, and collard greens). Broccoli, cauliflower, squash, zucchini, and cabbage last up to a week in the fridge so you should consume these later on (cabbage, squash, and zucchini can last up to two weeks).

Be aware of when your fruit and avocados have ripened so you eat them at the optimal time. A great tip: If you've got a bunch of fruit or avocados that is ripening quickly and you don't think you'll eat it all in time, throw everything you have into the fridge. This will immediately halt the ripening process and give you time so your produce doesn't go bad. Always remember that you can also freeze ripened fruit for use in smoothies and desserts (more on this to come), so you never need to worry about buying too much of it.

Stock up on citrus fruits (grapefruit, orange, and lemon), apples, carrots, and celery. These last very long in the fridge so you can buy them in bulk. You should always have a pantry fully stocked with onions, which go great in sautés, baked dishes, and salads. Onions will last you a couple of months without having to be refrigerated.

Save yourself time and keep yourself straight by heading to the store and stocking up. Your lean body depends on it.

Grains: The Gateway to Lean

In addition to having your home stocked with produce, you need to make sure you have whole grains on hand at all times. Contrary to mainstream diets that advise you to load up on protein instead of carbohydrates, the lean and functional body is based on a diet of healthy, whole grain (not wheat!) carbs.

As you learned in Part I, getting lean entails becoming an athlete—which means eating and working out, *not* exercising and dieting. If you're following the athletic mentality, whole grains should be the foundation of your diet.

The grains that will facilitate the lean body are single-ingredient, slow energy-releasing (and ideally, organic) grains such as buckwheat (kasha), brown rice, wild rice, steel cut oats, and quinoa (brown rice pasta is also an option to include once in a while). Forget the breads, the wheat pastas, the tortillas, the white rices, and the pizza crusts.

Grains taste best when they're fresh and hot off the stove, but preparing them from scratch at every meal can be time-consuming and burdensome. Instead, prepare extra large portions and then refrigerate the leftovers. Cooked grains will last at least four days and you can heat them up quickly and easily (without using a microwave!) by laying them out on a plate and throwing hot, freshly sautéed or steamed vegetables directly on top.

With raw grains in your cupboard and cooked grains in your fridge, you'll never come home to an empty kitchen. Even if you run out of produce from your big weekly marketing, you can still pick up some fish, meat, or vegetables on your way home from work and combine these ingredients with grains to construct a full meal.

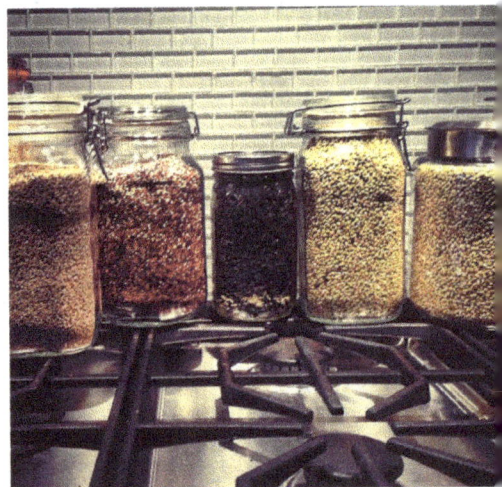

Grains will become a staple of your diet. From left to right: steel-cut oats, red quinoa, black rice, and raw kasha (buckwheat).

You can designate one day (I use Sunday) to prepare several batches of different grains for the week. Having multiple varieties at your disposal will be ideal, given that you probably don't want to eat quinoa for five days straight. You can bring your cooked grains with you for lunch, or simply have them ready and accessible when you get home.

Start today by stocking up on whole grains and getting that water boiling. Buckwheat is the quickest to prepare (about 5-6 minutes), quinoa and steel cut oats need more time (10 minutes or so), and brown and wild rice take the longest (approximately 25-30 minutes).

Stock Up on Nuts, Dried Fruit, and Dark Chocolate

Dried fruit and nuts are an integral part of the lean body diet and you should eat them often—either as a snack, in a salad, or on a dessert plate.

The dried fruit and nuts you purchase should be pure, meaning they shouldn't contain any added oil, sugar, or preservatives. You need to be extra careful with your purchases because many of these products do contain such additives.

Always check the ingredients list. When it comes to dried fruit, you need to be particularly careful with cranberries, pineapple, currants, papaya, cherries, blueberries and apricots, because they often contain unwanted ingredients.

The dried fruits I eat are figs, dates, prunes, and raisins. I buy the dates and the figs in bulk, and the prunes and raisins are "Newman's Own" brand. While Newman's Own offers a pure variety of prunes and raisins, their dried cranberries contain added cane sugar and sunflower oil, as does the "berry blend." Even if a brand sells one good product, you must always check labels on the others.

The nuts I usually eat are walnuts, Brazil nuts, and pecans. I buy these in bulk either online or in the local market. With nuts, you need to be on the lookout for added oils. Avoid peanuts—they contain unhealthy saturated fatty-acids and will hinder your lean body success.

A great compliment to your nuts and dried fruit is 85% dark chocolate. By eating dark chocolate, you'll avoid added sugar (the dried fruit will already be sweet enough) while still gaining the antioxidants and flavonols present in cacao.

A couple more points of note: (1) Pre-packaged and pre-assembled trail mixes almost always contain added sugar and oil. You should buy your dried fruit and nuts separately and make your own trail mix; (2) Be on the lookout for added preservatives such as sulfur dioxide, which are present in many dried fruit options; (3) Eat whole nuts and avoid nut butters—nut butters will make you gain weight.

One great tip is to use whole dates as a "spread" instead of sugary and preservative-filled jams. Make sure to buy dates with the *pits still inside*, as these are the juiciest. If you're eating a piece of toasted Mestemacher or Dimpflmeier bread, take out the pit and thinly spread the date across with your fingers.

Snack on Carrots, Celery, and Apples

Learning to snack in the right way will allow you to maximize your lean body efforts—and so you need to make sure you're eating nutritious foods when hunger comes on between meals.

The snack industry today is worth billions of dollars—and this makes sense. The snack foods being offered out there are addicting, they're widely available, they're convenient to eat, and they never spoil. Unhealthy snacks are offered at every turn you take—whether you're in a high school hallway or a gas station on the way to work. If you don't have healthy alternatives on hand, it's almost impossible to avoid these temptations.

Carrots, celery, and apples are easy and quick to wash and take with you on the go. Even more, you can stock up on these at home without having to worry because they stay fresh for a long time in the fridge.

Throw the carrots and celery into a Ziploc bag like you're a little kid again. It's better to snack on vegetables whenever possible because they will keep your blood sugar level stable. Plus, if you're having a desire to eat raw vegetables, you know that you're experiencing true hunger and not some craving. Fruits are best to snack on during or after workouts because they provide you with quick energy in the form of carbohydrates, not to mention added hydration (you will learn in the next chapter why replacing sports drinks with fruit is an effective, lean body building strategy).

When buying carrots, avoid baby carrots and choose the regular version. Baby carrots are mechanically processed into their "baby" state and some companies even use chlorine to wash them. Better to just get the real thing and wash it yourself in plain water.

Once you've mastered your carrot and celery snacking, you can move on to more advanced vegetable snacks such as cucumbers, raw broccoli, and radishes.

Run Your Dishwasher Once Per Day

Once you're on your way to mastering your nutrition and getting leaner, you'll soon notice that you're spending a lot more time in the kitchen.

A great gauge to see if you're staying true to the lean body diet is to ask yourself: Am I running my dishwasher regularly? If the answer is yes, odds are you're getting leaner, healthier, and closer to a mastered physical self. If the answer is no, you'd better start reassessing your routines.

Your dishwasher should be running at least once every couple days. Be proud of yourself if you can hear the faint hymn of your faithful, robotic friend in the background.

When you're on a routine of cooking your own food, scrubbing plates, and loading and unloading the dishwasher, you'll begin to come to terms with the fact that leaning down isn't easy work. It requires heart, dedication, and persistence. Getting there certainly isn't glamorous (you already know about "getting down and dirty"), but once you arrive you'll see that your efforts were all worth it.

CHAPTER 7
MASTER
YOUR FRUIT

Start Freezing Your Fruit

When you eat fruit, you need to make sure it's fully ripened. "Ripening" is a chemical change that increases levels of naturally occurring fruit sugars and antioxidants. Not only will it taste better, but you'll reap the fruit's full nutritional benefit.

Buying a variety of fruit and allowing it to sit out in your kitchen and ripen is the way to go, but sometimes it can be difficult to gauge how much you should purchase. You should err on the side of buying too much because leftover ripened fruit is great to freeze and store for future use in smoothies and desserts.

Eating a frozen pear or nectarine is like having a healthy sorbet (make sure to let it sit out for a few minutes so you don't break your teeth)—and as you get used to eating these frozen fruits, they'll taste even better! Having a wide range of frozen fruit accessible will enable you to create delicious fruit and vegetable smoothies on a whim.

The most important piece of frozen fruit is the frozen banana. Not only will the frozen banana be the foundation of your fruit and vegetable smoothie, but it will also be able to quench your sweet tooth like none other. Next time you find yourself fantasizing about a pint of Ben and Jerry's, reach for a frozen banana instead (more to come on preparing the healthy dessert).

It's important that *you are freezing your own fruit*, and not buying pre-packaged frozen fruit and berries. Buying pre-frozen fruit is certainly convenient, but since I began freezing my own, I can taste a world of difference (my own frozen fruit has significantly more flavor). Moreover, similar to pre-washed lettuce and carrots, many brands that sell frozen fruit wash their produce in chlorinated water, which in turn makes its way into your body.

I wonder how this fruit looks (and would taste) fresh before they freeze it to sell to you? It's likely the case that these berries, mangos, and peaches were rejects that wouldn't sell in the fresh produce market—yet repackaged as frozen, they're able to still bring in revenue from it.

Fruit and berries are cheaper in the summer time, so it's smart to freeze a bunch towards the latter summer months and store it for use throughout the fall. I usually do this for berries, and one night in late August I found myself alone on a Friday night at home, washing and cutting off the stems of a couple hundred strawberry packages well into the early morning hours. By the end of it, my freezer was stacked to the brim, and the supply lasted well into the final weeks of December.

Get Yourself a Blender

Introducing the fruit and vegetable smoothie into your daily routine will prove invaluable in your lean body quest.

Making a daily smoothie will right away up your fruit and veggie intake. Ultimately, you want to be eating these fruits and vegetables whole—not blended—as part of your meals, but the first step to getting there is through the smoothie (I myself started with the smoothie, so I can verify its effectiveness).

Vitamix is the top-of-the-line blender due to its high powered motor that liquefies everything—and I saved up to buy one over the course of several months. Vitamix baseline models begin at $300, so I would recommend starting with another cheaper brand, such as Ninja or KitchenAid.

The smoothies that you will be making are simple. The base of the smoothie will be the frozen banana (before freezing them, make sure they're fully ripened and peel the skin off). Your liquid base will be water.

As we discussed, you should also keep other frozen fruit available for use in the smoothie such as pears, mangos, nectarines, and peaches—and use these to supplement the banana. Sweet, frozen fruit will make the beverage cold and refreshing.

The vegetables to add are any mix of the following: carrot, celery, kale, beet, broccoli, and chard. You can also add fresh apple, grapefruit, and orange.

One other smoothie variation you can make that *doesn't include frozen banana* is beets, fresh ginger, grapefruit, and frozen pear or frozen apple. This is a delicious recipe, so try it out.

Drinking a smoothie alone will not be enough before a tough workout—you will need some grains to get yourself through. Smoothies should be consumed as a snack during the day, as a breakfast alternative on a day you're not working out, or as a refreshing post workout cooldown drink to hold you over until your next meal.

I started the transition to the lean body diet my senior year at Harvard, and I brought my Vitamix with me to Cambridge that fall semester. I stored the Vitamix in the dorm's communal kitchen and I was whipping up fresh Vitamix smoothies every day before classes. The kitchen was open to everyone and so I didn't have control over who used the blender while it was stored there. Aside from one student who misguidedly concocted a cake batter, nobody touched the blender during the entire year (thankfully). I also stored the fruits and vegetables in the communal fridge, but nobody seemed much interested in kale or broccoli either.

(I didn't have the time, preparation space, or even freezer space available to store frozen fruit, and so I was forced to drink these smoothies warm. They tasted horrible, but the experience makes me appreciate my chilled smoothies even more whenever I have them.)

Get a blender and start making some healthy smoothies. They will help you burst out of the gates in your path towards attaining the lean body and mastering your nutrition.

Creating the Healthy Dessert

Eating dessert shouldn't be an activity of guilt and wrongdoing but rather should be one of the most pleasurable and *healthy* activities that you do during the course of your day.

The first step to preparing the healthy dessert—like your other food—is to make sure that *you and only you* are preparing it. We've already touched on the ingredients involved—now all you need to do is assemble them.

Your desserts should include fresh or frozen fruit, berries, nuts, dried fruit, and 85% dark chocolate. Take a frozen banana (add some cinnamon) and sprinkle some raisins and walnuts on top. Create a plate of strawberries, blueberries, raspberries, Brazil nuts,

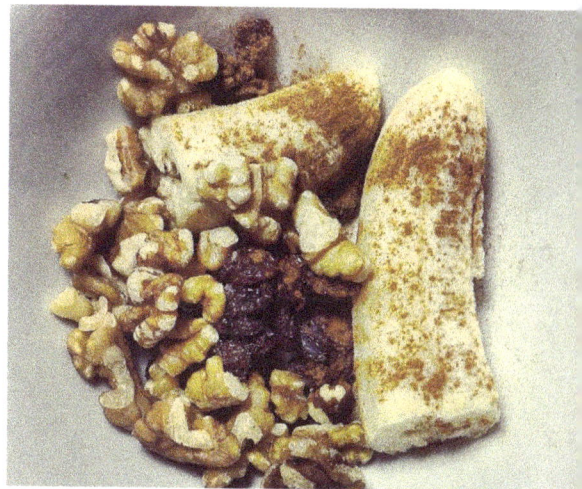

Frozen banana with cinnamon alongside raisins and walnuts. Frozen banana should be the base of your healthy dessert.

and dark chocolate. Treat yourself to a frozen pear with a side of figs. (Remember: when you're eating frozen fruit, allow it to thaw out for five minutes before eating. It will taste better and you won't risk cracking a tooth.)

The prevalent conception that sweets are bad for you is wrong—consuming sugar (natural sugar) is an integral and indispensable part of daily life. The body craves this sugar because it needs it—you just want to make sure it's the right kind.

Healthy, natural sugar can and should be eaten throughout the day, in addition to being consumed after meals as desserts. Part of your food preparation involves having a fresh apple or a bag of dates and walnuts with you at all times.

The next time your waiter offers you a crème brulee, tell him your healthy dessert is at home. It's time to start using your sweets to help you get leaner, and it's possible once you become your own dessert chef.

Get Your Citrus On

Eating citrus is part of building the lean body. Your home should always be stocked with lemons, oranges, and grapefruits, and given that these last for extended periods in the fridge (up to two months!), you shouldn't display any reserve when it comes to buying large amounts of them.

Lemon is a great addition to a cold glass of water and should be used regularly. Lemons provide many health benefits that include strengthening the immune system, promoting weight loss, and assisting in digestion. Even more, squeezing fresh lemon into your water will make you want to drink more, promoting a fully hydrated body. I usually have a glass of cold water with lemon right when I wake up.

Oranges and grapefruit are excellent options for breakfast and dessert, as well as snacks throughout the day. You want to eat these fruits whole, so don't just squeeze out the juice—consuming them whole will enable you to obtain the majority of their phytonutrients, which reside primarily in the pulp.

On days when I'm not working out, I'll often slice up a grapefruit and have that for breakfast (my first meal on off-days is usually an early lunch around 11 o'clock). Nothing beats downing a couple of chilled oranges after an intense workout—certainly beats a heavily processed, artificial "recovery"/protein drink.

Stock your fridge with some orange and yellow and benefit from the power of citrus in your life.

Forget Sports Drinks and Eat Fruit Instead

In building the lean body, water should be the only fluid you drink and all of your calories should be coming from food only (I consider the smoothie to qualify because the base of the drink is water and the rest consists of whole fruits and vegetables).

In order to do this, you must do away with the sports drinks, vitamin waters, and fitness waters. People looking to improve their health through exercise have been misled by marketing ploys to believe that sports drinks are actually good for them, and are beneficial for exercise and sports.

Don't be fooled. No matter which sports drink you choose—Gatorade, Powerade, or some low-calorie spinoff—it's going to be processed and it's going to contain unhealthy ingredients. These drinks contain dyes, preservatives, syrups, sweeteners, and artificial additives. True sportsmen concerned about their performance and health aren't putting these drinks into their bodies (and if they tell you otherwise, it's because they've signed a multi-million

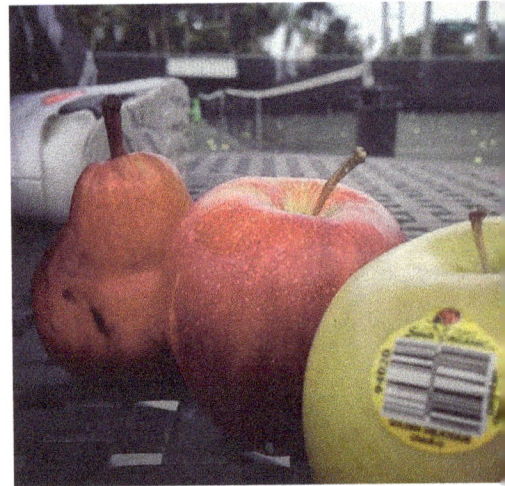

Always bring fruit with you to your training. Fuel yourself with fresh fruit and mineral water during your workouts and watch the lean body take form.

dollar contract). The real high-level athletes are using carefully crafted concoctions that their elite trainers or national sports federations have developed specifically for them and their performance needs.

Start bringing fresh fruit to your workout and do away with the sports drinks. When you're thirsty, drink water, and when you need a carbohydrate boost, eat an apple or pear. Don't eat the entire piece of fruit at once—instead take some bites over the course of a ten minute period. This will work to steadily elevate your blood sugar level and keep it there. Fruit is great to consume during and after a workout because it provides instant carbohydrates and energy that the body can absorb quickly.

In addition to fueling your body with fruit, you should aim to drink mineral water during your workouts. Drinking mineral water during a workout is like eating because the water is heavier and will make you feel full—you will be able to push through a multi-hour training session on a smaller food portion, without experiencing hunger. By directly replacing the minerals lost in your sweat, you will also find yourself drinking less too, thereby optimizing the functionality of your body because you won't be loaded down with excess fluid.

Drinking mineral water during workouts was one of the key realizations that enabled me to take my body to the next level of lean— and I had this epiphone when I was in Europe competing in tennis. Go to any snack bar at any European tennis club to buy water before a match, and it will always be mineral water. I soon noticed a huge difference in the way I was feeling: I was able to play many hours on the court without any hunger. It took me some time to connect the difference in performance to the mineral water, but once I did, I never went back.

In the United States, mineral water is almost impossible to come by (the only brand I've seen widely available is Evian, which is imported from France). Most water offered in America is either filtered or "spring," both of which have low mineral content. Before your next workout, eat a smaller portion of food, pick up a chilled bottle of Evian, and you will soon notice that you can go harder and longer on less.

CHAPTER 8
OPTIMIZE YOUR DIET

You Just Ate. How Do You Feel?

Perfecting your shopping cart is a process of trial and error. While I provide you with the blueprint of the lean body diet, you need to be able to gauge what's working for you and what's not. Paying close attention to the way your body feels, particularly after meals, will allow you to progress further than you ever could have imagined.

If the ingredients in your meal were healthy, nutritious, and fit well with your body, you should be feeling light after eating, and the meal should be absorbed fully in the stomach within 30-45 minutes.

If you've just eaten but you're unsure how you feel, head out for a light workout (ideally a run) after an hour. If the meal was proper, you should feel light, energized, and ready to push yourself. If the food is still in your chest or throat, you need to alter what you're eating or the portion size. If you feel weak, the proportion of grains to vegetables and fish/meat probably isn't optimal (correct this by increasing the amount of grains).

You should also pay attention to how you feel four or five hours after a meal. For example, if you feel swollen or are retaining too much fluid, you should down your salt intake. If you're heading for a run and feel heavy, you might have had too much meat on your plate.

Be sure you don't overeat. Eating natural, single-ingredient (and ideally, organic) foods will work to self-regulate your food consumption—it's nearly impossible to overeat foods like brown rice, broccoli, avocado, and fish. Even so, you always want to be aware of your portion size and make sure you don't overdo it.

Operate Flawlessly

Full effort and full execution are necessary to build the lean body. There's no middle ground and there's no halfway there if you want to get results—especially quick results. Either you're doing the right things or you're not.

Whenever I'm at the grocery store, I always look around at other people's shopping carts. Usually, what I see is a middle-ground assortment. Someone buying fresh fruit with frozen pizza. Another person buying fresh vegetables alongside Oreos and Doritos. Someone else buying organic popcorn. These people have the right intention in choosing "organic," or in trying to buy more vegetables or fruit—but they're still falling short of maximizing their efforts.

When you grocery shop, you should aim to buy raw, unprepared, unprocessed, whole, single-ingredient foods. Navigate the supermarket on the periphery and avoid the center aisles, which is where most of the pre-packaged, processed, and frozen food is offered. Buy fresh vegetables to steam and use in salads. Buy raw fish and lean meat. Stock up on raw, whole grains to boil on your stovetop. Fill your cupboards with nuts, dried fruit, and 85% dark chocolate.

Forget processed deli meats, as these generally contain preservatives and nitrites. Also, avoid nutrition bars and other packaged snacks and begin fueling your body with fresh fruit and raw vegetables instead. The pre-cut melon at the supermarket is usually jacked up in price; you're better off with some organic apples or bananas, which will save you money and do more for your health (nutrients leave the fruit when it's cut up and left to sit for long periods).

Eat Kasha

Brown rice and quinoa are well-known healthy whole grain options, but few are aware of kasha (buckwheat). Kasha should be a staple grain of your diet, so fill up your cart with some the next time you head to the market.

While I refer to kasha as a "grain," kasha is actually a fruit seed related to rhubarb and sorrel. Kasha is filling, quick-to-cook (it only needs 5-6 minutes on the stovetop), and high in both carbohydrates *and* protein. Due to kasha's high fiber content compared to brown rice (more than double), the body requires more time to digest it, in turn controlling hunger levels. In addition, kasha is a great way to top off a vegetarian meal because at nearly 6 grams of protein per cup, you will feel fully satiated without any added meat or fish.

Supermarkets offer kasha in two varieties: toasted and raw. When I first started preparing kasha, I was eating the raw variety, but have since transitioned to toasted kasha. Kasha is a staple of the Eastern European diet, and there is a Russian store near my house where I buy my favorite brand (imported from Russia), "Uvelka." Because kasha cooks so quickly, it's always my go-to when I come home from a workout—I can throw it on the stove to simmer before jumping into the shower. Within minutes, I have a hot plate of food that I can combine with a fresh salad, avocado, steamed vegetables and/or left-over fish or meat from dinner the night before. Be careful not to overcook your kasha, which I was doing for the first year before a Russian friend came for lunch and made me aware that cooked kasha should have a hardened consistency.

The obesity epidemic afflicting the United States today isn't by chance—the foods offered on our home soil are addicting, stimulating, and nutrition-free. It's a plain fact that very few Americans eat kasha on a regular basis. Start bypassing the dangers of the American food landscape by filling up your cart with this Eastern European mainstay. It's one of the best kept secrets out there.

Replace Meat With Fish

To attain the lean body, you will need to down your red meat and poultry consumption, and up your fish intake.

Fish is high in protein, and it's packed with essential nutrients and omega-3 fatty acids—ingredients that will work wonders for your fitness and possibly save you from heart disease in the process.

Transitioning to eating fish instead of other animal meats will lean you down right away. Since limiting my chicken and red meat intake, I've become ten pounds lighter. My chest and stomach melted away and the muscles in my limbs finally saw the light of day.

When you buy fish, you should be getting "wild caught" and not farm-raised. Wild fish is the only animal still out there not subjected to the horrendous practices of the modern farming industry. When you eat wild fish, you're getting an animal that was living in its natural habitat, moving about freely, and consuming the things it was naturally intended to—not corn feed, artificial colors, or antibiotics.

You must be extra cautious when purchasing fish to make sure you're getting the right product. The other day at the supermarket fish counter I noticed a piece of bright red salmon being sold, a hue so striking you had to see it to believe it. It turned out that this salmon selection was not only farm-raised, but it was also *color enhanced through feed.* You should be on the lookout for products that seem unnatural or "too good to be true," and always request product information before making a purchase.

Fish is easy to prepare and it cooks quickly. You can steam it or throw it into the oven, both of which take less than 15 minutes depending on the thickness of the piece.

Eating fish often means you need to watch your methyl mercury consumption. Methyl mercury is an organic compound that accumulates in fish during the course of their lifetime—and fish that live longer and stand higher up on the food chain contain more mercury. You should be eating fish no more than two times per week and aim to consume smaller fish that contain less mercury. The two primary fish types in my own diet are sardines and flounder—which I've intentionally selected due to their low mercury levels. Salmon and cod, although they contain slightly more mercury, are also great options that I include too. Refrain from eating tuna, marlin, swordfish, and grouper, which contain high mercury levels.

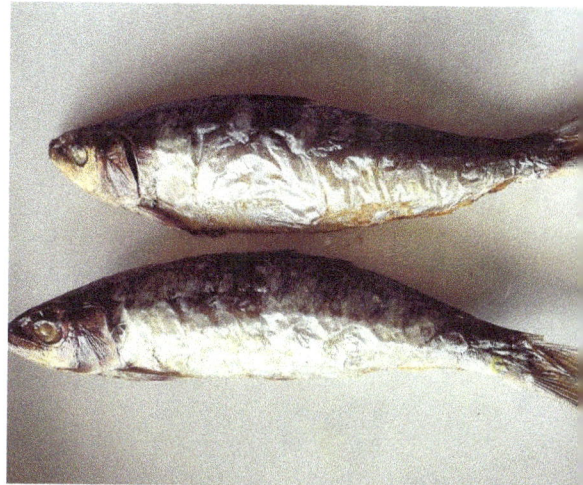

Roasted sardines, which are low in mercury and high in protein and omega-3 fatty acids. You can order frozen sardines online and they cook quickly in the oven.

Steam Vegetables

Leaning down involves getting into the habit of regularly preparing steamed vegetables at meals. Steamed vegetables are healthy, they're fast to cook, and they're filling. Even more, they're digested quickly and easily so you can head out for a workout soon after.

Steaming is a great cooking option because you'll avoid added oils that might have been included in a sauté. Also, steaming requires minimal prep and clean-up time, which is ideal if you're rushed or if you're particularly famished when you get home.

If you aren't experienced in the kitchen, start by steaming broccoli, cauliflower, and red cabbage. Not only are these some of the healthiest vegetables out there, but they're also some of the most filling.

These three vegetables stay fresh for up to a week in the fridge (cabbage up to two weeks) and they're easy to wash. One great tip when it comes to broccoli prepartion: you can eat the stem as well

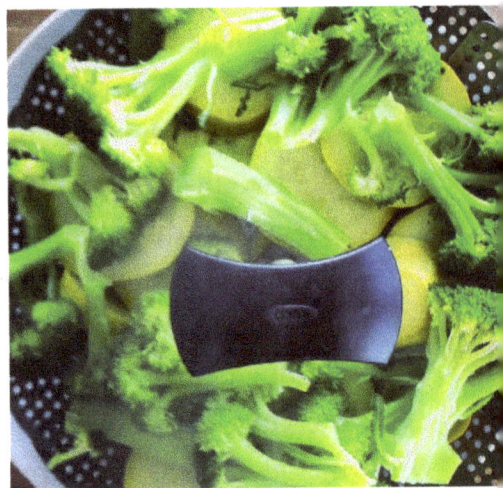

Steamed broccoli and squash. Steaming your vegetables is not only one of the healthiest ways to prepare them, but it's also the quickest. Buy a steaming basket so you can steam your veggies on the stovetop in a large pot (make sure the steaming basket sits above the boiling water).

by peeling the outermost layer, which is tough and inedible, with a sharp knife. Once peeled, the broccoli stem will need about 3 or 4 minutes of extra cooking time than the flowery head, but it's worth it—the stem is both filling and nutritious!

Once you've become a more expert steamer, you can branch into leafy greens (chard, collard, kale, bok choy), which necessitate more extensive prep time and quicker consumption from the time of purchase (leafy greens wilt within a few days).

Assuming you've stored some pre-cooked grains in the fridge to last you the week, you can avoid heating these grains up in the microwave by placing the hot, steamed veggies over a plate of cold grains. Let it sit for a couple minutes and voilà—you've got a hot, healthy meal in minutes.

Be sure not to overcook the vegetables because doing so will detract from the flavor and destroy the full nutritional benefit. Rule of thumb: undercooking is better than overcooking. The broccoli head will require the least amount of time (3 minutes), and the cabbage, cauliflower, and broccoli stem will need slightly more (6-7 minutes).

Exercise and Appetite

The final step in optimizing your diet, once you've secured the best ingredients and know how to prepare them, is to effectively balance your exercise and eating.

Exercise is vital to regulate your appetite and feel what type of "fuel" your body needs. Assuming you're working out properly (explained in Part I), you'll be burning off excess stored energy and heat, which will work to recalibrate your body—and it's this recalibration that will enable you to gauge your hunger.

You never want to eat a meal because "it's time" to do so. You should have a clear understanding of your hunger before sitting down to eat, and this can only be done through regular workouts.

In my own experience, whenever I complete an extended training session I can feel my hunger with precision. The hunger is clear and the appetite pressing.

When I take a day off, on the other hand, my hunger becomes dulled. The hunger on an off day comes about in the form of a light-headedness (or if I'm reading or writing, in the form of dampened mental clarity), whereas the hunger on a workout day hits me at the core of my stomach.

Follow these two easy steps to master your appetite through exercise: (1) Make sure you're doing some type of exercise—even if it's just ten minutes—before breakfast and dinner. I would recommend running, but in the beginning it doesn't much matter, just get the body moving. (2) After you complete your exercise, wait 20-30 minutes for your appetite to come on—and listen carefully to it. Determine whether your body needs a larger piece of fish/meat or a heavier serving of grains. Pay attention to how hungry you feel in order to consume the proper portion.

Start using exercise to gauge your appetite—this will prove instrumental in your quest to build the lean body.

Arrange Your Meals and Workouts To Avoid Caffeine

Effectively balancing your meals and workouts isn't just useful in curbing your appetite, it will also allow you to stay alert and energized throughout the day without having to consume caffeine.

Getting lean entails ridding the body of compromisers so that it can function independently and fluidly. The macchiatos, Red Bulls, Monster Energy drinks, 5-Hour Energy shots, pre-workout supplements, and other caffeine-jacked substances will counter your efforts towards buildling a crisply functioning, lean, healthy body. While caffeine may give you a momentary burst or even dampen your appetite in the moment, the long-term effects will numb your connection to your body.

Caffeine is one of the most prevalent and widespread addictions out there, yet we don't readily regard it as such. What would happen if the country's supply of caffeine dwindled, for a day or even a week, forcing people to function without it? A majority would be rendered inoperant. They would be walking around like zombies, probably falling asleep mid-day on the sidewalks.

Caffeine is a powerful substance that hooks you in quickly, forcefully, and unsuspectingly—and once you're in, there's no getting out. Times when I've drank coffee for several consecutive days, and then gone off it, I've felt lethargic and mentally-clouded in the days following. The withdrawal hit me right away, even as a non-coffee drinker.

Coffee isn't just bad because it's addicting, but it also produces inflammation inside the body. It zaps out energy levels (after the initial adrenaline wears off), creates a physical and psychological dependency, and alters the Circadian rhythm.

Optimizing your diet (and life) involves using the food you're eating—and the way you structure your eating schedule combined with exercise—to keep you awake and in-tune throughout your day.

Before your breakfast you should be going for a run, as we've already addressed. This will wake you up right away *without coffee*, and if you eat a large breakfast around 9 o'clock or 10, your sugar levels (and your alertness) will stay elevated until the early afternoon.

As soon as you feel yourself fading around 12 or 1, head for another light workout session. Working out a second time—even for a short period—will wake you up and get your body ready to efficiently take in your lunch.

Lunch should be eaten around 2 o'clock—and you should aim to push that meal as late as possible to avoid an afternoon lull. If you eat later on, your blood sugar will stay high well into the late afternoon hours. If you still feel yourself getting tired, eat a piece of fresh fruit to reinvigorate you.

Timing your meals properly, using exercise to re-energize you, and taking advantage of the sugar boost from fruit when necessary will enable you to transition away from coffee and into an addiction-free and Feel-Good State.

PART III:
LEAN DOWN YOUR LIFE

CHAPTER 9
THE FEEL-GOOD STATE

The Feel-Good State

The Feel-Good State is a centerpiece of *The Lean Body Manual* because in order to get lean, you need to feel good in your body. When you've reached the Feel-Good state, you will be in-tune with your body and able to hear the signs it's giving you (for example, you will have an accurate gauge on your hunger and you will know when it's time to stretch out your lower back).

Reaching the Feel-Good State is no small feat, and your daily efforts should be focused on making you feel the best you can physically and mentally. Much of what's being offered out there—whether it's unhealthy food, nightlife and alcohol, or some exercise gimmick—counters your good feelings. Therefore, it's crucial to identify the specific ingredients in your life that make you feel good and then work to secure these ingredients on a regular basis. The path to reaching the Feel-Good State is different for everyone, and so you need to know yourself well.

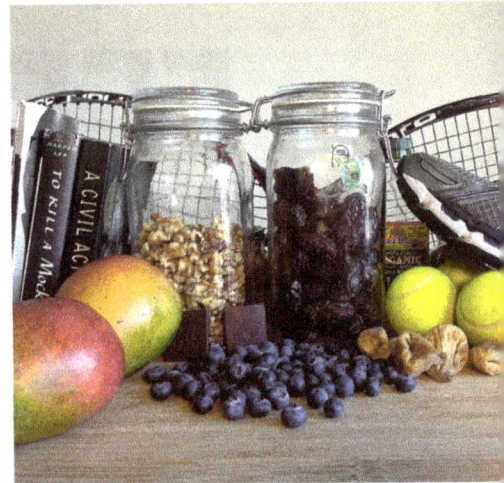

The Feel-Good State comes from eating healthy food, pursuing a consistent exercise regimen, and grounding the mind through healthy mental routines.

Proper nutrition, a consistent exercise regimen, and a clear mind are all universal requirements for the Feel-Good State. A proper support network of people who care about you and who have your best interests in mind is also important.

Building the lean body and finding the Feel-Good State maintain a dynamic and symbiotic relationship. If you're getting leaner and fitter, odds are you're going to feel good. If you're feeling good, you will in turn be able to get the most out of your workouts and stay injury-free.

Start to look inside yourself and get in touch with your body. Ask yourself—how do I feel right now? How can I feel better? The only way to master your Feel-Good State is to look inwards and think about what's helping you and what's hurting.

Prioritize Your Physical and Mental Health

The process of getting lean is grounded in the health of your body and mind. We've already addressed many strategies in Parts I and II for securing your physical health, but that's only half the battle. You must also work diligently to keep the mind healthy too.

While the body and mind are robust in many ways, their health should never be taken for granted. Just like you manage your physical wellbeing by stretching out a muscle or altering your training equipment, you need to adjust your lifestyle to maintain a healthy mind. If you're suffering from chronic anxiety, fatigue or depression, you must analyze what's causing this and make a change. Think about your environment as well. Getting out of a mentally or physically oppressive situation early on will prevent you from suffering long term damage, either in the form of a physical injury or mental handicap like depression.

Always fight to protect your Feel-Good State. Don't compromise on your physical and mental health if you don't have to. We are nothing more than our bodies and minds, and if we don't take care of them, they won't take care of us. Getting lean and fit is more than aesthetics—it's about adopting a sound approach to life, where you're actively caring for yourself and protecting your best interest.

Find Passion

Passion is the single most important ingredient for securing your Feel-Good State. A passionate person is fully invested and engaged—in body, mind, and spirit. To be fully engaged in your pursuits—in such a way that nothing else enters your mind while you're following them—is the goal.

Ideally, you should be waking up every day and looking forward to what you're doing. Even in the pursuit of the lean body, you need to be 100% present. Convince yourself that getting lean is your passion. By continuing to invest in yourself and in the process, you will soon find yourself enjoying your workouts, your new meal plan, and the transformation you will soon experience. Sure, every moment might not be pleasant, but pushing through adversity is necessary to get where you want. A few moments of discomfort will be negligible in the scope of pursuing your dreams and accomplishing your goals.

Take a moment and think about your weekly schedule. How can I be more present? How can I rework my days to better incorporate the things I love? What adjustments can I make to have more energy and focus? These are a few critical questions to ask in optimizing your routines and arriving at your Feel-Good State.

In identifying passion, you must understand your goals, priorities, and inner self. Figure out what drives you at the core of your being. You might need to meditate on this topic in order to purge some insights about your direction and life choices. Keep a journal. Jot down notes throughout the day in your smart phone or planner. If something comes to mind at work or class, send an email to yourself. The process will take time, but it will be rewarding once you arrive. The ultimate objective is to find peace within yourself so you can move along in a worthwhile and valuable direction— one that isn't influenced by external

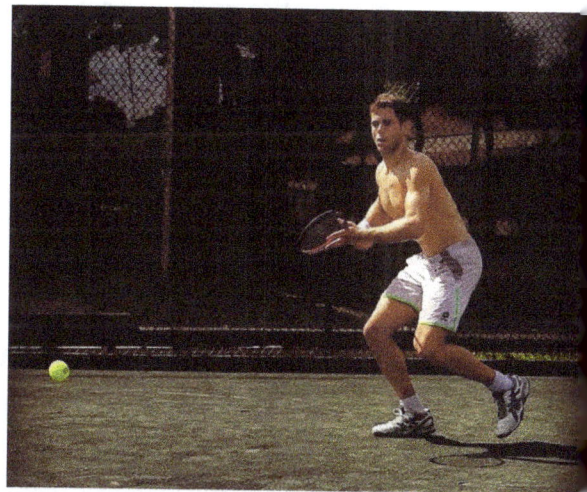

My passion for tennis has allowed me to find grounding in my life at large. Tennis has led me to a healthy, productive, and fulfilling life.

pressure or a misplaced desire to conform to some mold. To achieve your biggest dreams, you will need to become an independent thinker and actor.

The pursuit of passion works to ground the mind—which in turn secures prolonged mental health. If you're incorporating what you love into your life, something that arouses and invigorates your body and mind (even if it's only for an hour each day), the possibility of you becoming mentally compromised will diminish significantly. Having the ability to immerse yourself fully in a pursuit, routine, or activity is a huge asset. You can always return to this interest when times are tough, and use it to re-elevate you when things go wrong.

Identify what excites you and pursue it will full force. When you live life with invested emotion and an integrated spirit, your Feel-Good State will always be close.

Use Your Time and Money Wisely

The Feel-Good State involves using your money wisely, specifically to promote your physical and mental wellbeing. Time is your most precious asset, and so the money you take in from time spent at work, along with the time you have free away from your job and other responsibilities, should be targeted to assist you in building a healthy body and mind.

Think objectively when it comes to your purchases. Never invest in quick-fix guarantees or marketing gimmicks that propose farfetched outcomes. Forget the new smoothie diet in the informercial. Scroll past the online promo for that complicated looking ab contraption (it won't get you a six-pack). Never mind the designer hand-bag and shoes—they won't turn you into the talk of the town (but a lean body will!). Fleeting, superficial, non-enduring products won't get you where you want—only hard work done in the right way, where your body and mind are grounded.

Instead of buying an expensive watch or blowing your cash on a fancy cruise, put your money towards new running sneakers, a massage, or some fresh vegetables. Use your savings in the bank to have more time—to exercise, stretch out, meditate, read an interesting book, or prepare a healthy meal. Time is money, so make your money work for you by giving you more free moments to pursue your Feel-Good State.

Avoid the black hole of empty commercial promises. Get smart by ensuring that your consumption and free time are targeted.

Take a Break When You Need One

If you've been following a strict workout and diet plan consistently for many months, it's always smart to take a break. Building the lean body and securing the Feel-Good State take time, and you want to be sure not to burn out. Treat yourself to a meal out. Meditate in the park one afternoon. Take an afternoon to organize your living space. Spend Sunday with friends.

The human body and mind aren't machines. If you've made a great deal of progress within a compressed period of time, it's crucial for your health and longevity to put your efforts on hold so you can recharge and revitalize.

In my own experience, there were many times when I should have taken a break but didn't. Even though I could feel myself getting more and more tired with each passing day, I kept true to my routine. This harmed me in the long run because I burned out and needed many weeks to get myself going again.

It's important to distinguish between fatigue that you can push through, and fatigue that's telling you it's time to back off. Making the distinction isn't easy, but with some experience you will soon understand how to gauge these feelings. I myself needed to make this mistake once or twice before I learned.

Never underestimate the value of a "Feel-Good Support Network," so be sure to surround yourself with caring, intelligent people. Pay close attention to the advice and recommendations your supporting actors give you. If you have the right people behind you, they will have your best interests in mind and will be able to assist you in managing your outputs. During the last several years, I've made some like-minded friends who I can speak freely with about my fitness and life goals—and this has made all the difference. Don't be afraid to share your thoughts with others you are close with, and be sure to help your friends and family sort through their internal struggles as well.

When you're pushing yourself to your limits, you're more prone to injury—whether physical injury or a compromised mind. It's the times when you're on edge that you need to be particularly careful. Fight for your goals but protect your Feel-Good State in the process.

Maximize Your Surrounding Energy

Finding the Feel-Good State involves using the energies around you in the best way possible. The three types of energy that you need channel are (1) positive, (2) neutral, and (3) negative.

If you've managed to foster a network around you that's promoting positive energy, congratulations—this is no easy feat. This positive support network— the Feel Good Support Network—will prove invaluable in your quest to lead a lean and productive life. Soak in this energy. Breathe it in. Allow it to circulate throughout your entire organism. Try to

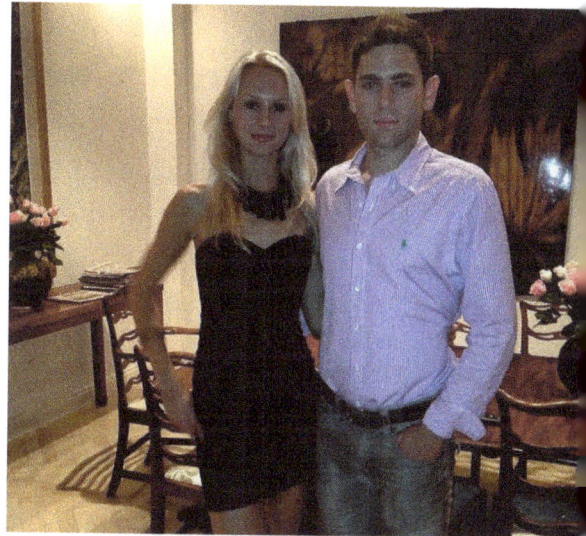

My fiancée Lyuda is part of my Feel Good Support Network. Without positive support behind you, it will be impossible for you to accomplish your fitness and life goals.

feed off of it so as to boost your own positivity. A Feel Good Support Network is an incredible resource, so make the most of it.

If you are surrounded by neutral energies, try to convert these into positive ones. If there is someone sitting next to you in the office or classroom who isn't particularly positive or negative, try to make an effort towards him or her. Ask about the person's day or weekend. Offer up some of your fresh fruit and vegetable smoothie. Share some of the lean body strategies you've learned in this book. Converting as many neutral energies into positive ones will enable you to feel your best and achieve the maximum progress in the long run.

Lastly, if you are surrounded by negative energies, it is actually possible to use these to your benefit. In many cases, people envy those who are enjoying success and reaping the benefits of hard work (so if you're getting leaner, don't be surprised if you experience some pushback). This jealous energy is often displayed through negativity. First of all, know that if you find this type of energy directed towards you, it isn't necessarily a bad thing—this could often signify that you're moving in the right direction. By perceiving jealousy as affirmation that you're achieving your goals, you can use it to encourage you even further. Pump yourself up in your next lean body workout, and benefit from even greater results.

CHAPTER 10
COMMIT

Leaning Down: A Long-Term Approach

While you will surely get results in the first few weeks of your lean body program, you must remember that building the lean body is a long-term endeavor. Your goal should be to make progress now and well into the future. Use *The Lean Body Manual* to build a healthy, fit, and enduring body for life!

Those who build truly fit and enduring bodies invest years of persistent efforts and unwavering dedication to their goals. You need to make sure you're doing the right things day in and day out, and continuing to do so even when the environment or circumstances prove difficult. Keep in mind that everything we have discussed thus far must be absorbed and understood within the time frame of years, not months and not days.

This book provides you with the foundation for a sustainable regimen towards attaining your fitness and nutrition goals. It's not a quick fix, it's a lifestyle change. If you want to achieve lasting results, you will need to display dedication and determination for the long-run. You need to committ fully and understand that temporary progress is far from permanent change. Start to get in the right mindset so that you can begin building your body properly and follow through with your routines for the rest of your life.

Invest in the Process

A widespread problem that prevents many people from reaching their full potential is that they don't invest in the process. When it comes to leaning down, you may very well hate every single workout you do, at least in the beginning. But you need to trick yourself—*convince yourself*—that you're loving every minute of it (this is not easy to do, but it's a skill you need to learn).

In order to lean down, you can't be thinking about end results. You need to be invested in the everyday moments that get you there. Don't look at the clock and don't think about the pain. Focus on the next stride, the next pushup, or the next healthy meal preparation. Embrace the process and the work that's moving you towards your goals.

I once overheard a girl telling her friend, "I can't wait until I'm thin because once I'm thin and I have a boyfriend, I can eat whatever I want." This is the perfect representation of the *wrong* mentality.

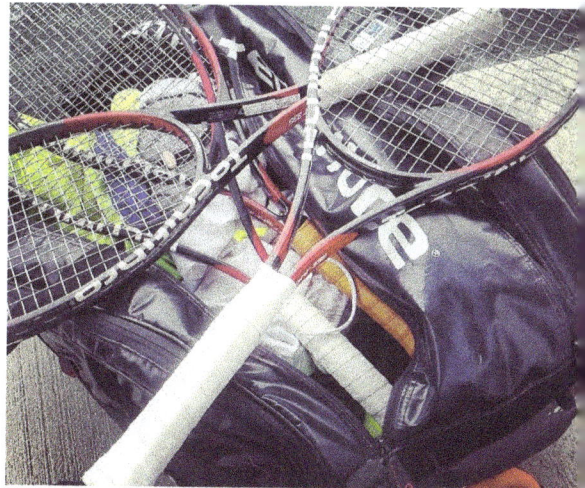

The process never stops, so invest yourself for the long haul. I'm still playing tennis nearly every day.

The process never stops. Once you get to your final destination, you need to work to stay there. Whether it's a lean body, a top-10 ranking on the ATP Tour, a CEO position at a Fortune 500 company, or getting a boyfriend (*and keeping one!*), achieving your goals doesn't mean you can then back off. You need to keep pushing so you stay there.

Note the phrase: "I can't wait." If you ever find yourself using this phrase in a context other than "I can't wait to get into my next workout" or "I can't wait to prepare a healthy dinner," you must take a step back and reassess. You can and must wait. Anything worthwhile only comes through struggle. And it takes time. As long as you know you're investing in the right choices everday, the results will come.

It's simple: (1) Invest yourself, even if you have to trick yourself you're invested; (2) Work hard and don't expect instant results; (3) Think long-run change and progress—*not* short-run burst followed by decline.

Extend Your Life Through Sports

While renting an apartment last year in Boca Raton, Florida, I met an affable neighbor—David—who appeared at first glance to be in his late 60s or early 70s. David is an exuberant man, and times when I saw him around the building he was always engaging with other residents or building staff.

At one point in the year I started to play tennis at a new facility, and the first morning I arrived there, David was playing on the court next to me. I had no idea he played tennis, and we soon got to talking.

David explained that he plays tennis five days a week for an hour and a half, always beginning bright and early at eight o'clock. David then informed he wasn't the age I suspected—*he is 88 years old!* I couldn't believe it, and not just because of how he looks. David was playing tennis every day in the full humidity of a Florida summer, with temperatures reaching well over 90 degrees.

As I spoke with David more, I learned that he first picked up a tennis racquet at the age of sixteen while growing up in Casablanca, Morocco, where his family ran a small hotel. David went on to have a long and successful career in the hospitality industry, and at whatever hotel he was stationed, he would always continue to develop his tennis game by playing at the hotel courts with colleagues or the teaching pros.

David's love for tennis propelled him to continue playing the game throughout the course of his life. Now, at 88, he looks, acts, and maintains the same energy as a man in the peak of his prime. In my conversations with David, I could tell that his mind was sharper than ever, as he could recall every relevant event in his life down to the exact day.

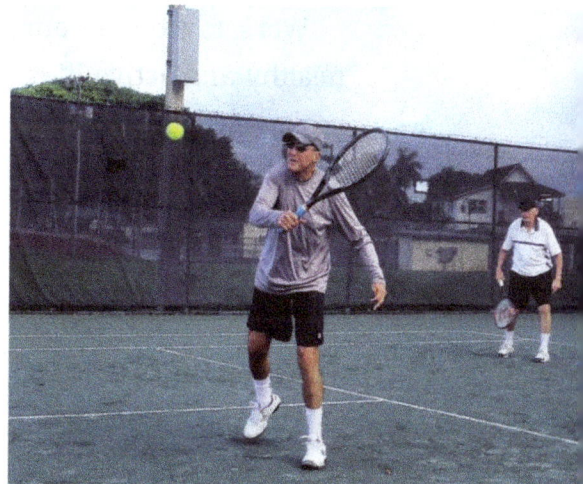

My 88 year-old neighbor David hitting a backhand volley. He has benefitted from a healthy body and sharp mind due to his commitment to staying active and playing sports.

David attributed his healthy body, crisp mind, and overall robust nature to the fact that he plays tennis every day. David explained, "After I play tennis in the morning, I'm ready to start my day and I know it's going to be a good one. Competing every day and staying active is what's keeping me healthy, feeling good, and enabling me to enjoy the uncompromised lifestyle that I now have."

The lifestyles of most people David's age are certainly burdened in some way—be it an ailing hip or a cloudy mind. But David is able to live a full, active, and engaged life because a daily routine of sports has kept him healthy and strong. He doesn't seem to be slowing down anytime soon—his routine of morning tennis will likely provide him with a high quality of life for many years to come.

Work to extend your life—and the quality of your life—through a healthy and active lifestyle. Identify what drives you in the physical realm—whether it's yoga, tennis, running, swimming, or biking—and then follow it. Use the diet and fitness advice in this book to further catapult you towards long-term health.

Ushering Out the Distractions

The lean lifestyle means using your time effectively and avoiding distractions that will zap out your energy. In order to push through your workouts and stick to your healthy meal plan, you need all of your reserves. Don't waste your precious personal resources: time, energy, focus.

Spend free moments in your day making a plan of action for your lean body program. Visualize your next workout. Note what you need to pick up at the grocery store. Adjust your iPod soundtrack for your next run. Stretch out your legs and arms if you feel tight.

When you're at the office or in the classroom, give your full focus to the task at hand. If you're able to become more efficient during these moments, you will get more done and then have extra time to allocate towards working out and eating healthfully. Plus, you'll have a clear mind because you'll have completed the work you needed to.

In this day and age, with a distraction everywhere you turn, it's even more crucial that you constantly reboot and refocus yourself. Take extra measures to ensure you're present in each moment. Block Facebook on your computer. Leave your phone behind when you head to work out. Make a shopping list of healthy choices before you head to the grocery store so you don't find yourself wandering.

The lean lifestyle is all about ushering out the distractions and the time wasting. Every moment is precious, particularly free time outside of work or school because this is when you can restore health in your body and invest in your fitness.

Momentum

Building momentum is crucial for leaning down. You need to be engaged in the proper routines consistently and for a long period of time, there's no other way to do it.

Whether it's your nutrition, exercise, or lean lifestyle, building momentum involves putting your head down and investing. Whenever you are able to foster *some* momentum, however little it is, you need to latch onto it and convert it into more.

Let's use the analogy of a tennis match to understand why momentum is so important and why it can mean the difference between reaching your goals and not. If you're building momentum in a tennis match, winning point after point and game after game, there's going to be little hope for your opponent. The score and the momentum are on your side.

Yet momentum is fragile, in both tennis and life. Even though you may be winning by a landslide, as soon as your opponent claims a few points in a row, no matter what the score is, he's going to gain some belief. This belief will lead

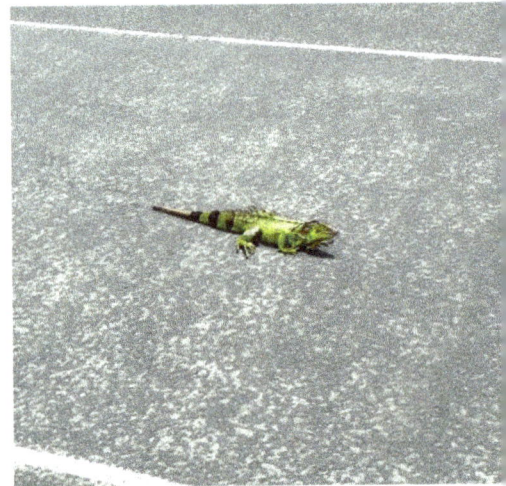

This iguana knows about the importance of momentum. I see him at the courts every day following through with his lean body fitness program.

him to win even more rallies, and very quickly steal the momentum over to his side. Before you know it, the score is even.

You often hear people say that a tennis match is decided by a few points. There's truth to this statement because there are momentum-changing points in a match—points that unequivocally shift momentum to one player or the other. Make the most of your momentum in two ways: (1) Once you've gained momentum, work to build off of it to create even more. (2) Ride out your momentum fully until you've reached your goals.

The first bits of momentum are always the hardest to build. As soon as you find yourself making progress, recognize this and keep pushing. Riding out your momentum "fully" is difficult, especially if you're putting forth a long term effort. But you'll certainly notice big changes along the way. Stay motivated and stay invested. Don't accept your current progress as the final destination.

Getting lean is like the clichéd "snowball effect." The more forward momentum you build, the faster your snowball of lean-ness will grow. When your snowball of lean-ness grows, it will in turn accelerate faster and grow even more.

In all of this, never focus on the results. Concentrate on the everyday tasks at hand. Once you arrive, you'll know it.

Reflect on Your Efforts

At the end of a training block (I would consider this to be every 4-6 weeks), you must sit yourself down to reflect on your lean body efforts and determine what you can improve. Analyze your struggles and successes, and use your realizations to modify your program for the future. By taking the time to reflect, you are investing in yourself and your long-term growth.

Pinpoint the routines that worked for you, along with the habits that detracted from your progress. Determine what you could be doing better. Pat yourself on the back for jobs you did well. The only way to get lean and stay lean over is to be honest with yourself, so don't bullshit. You know yourself best—be truthful and realistic.

In addition to reflecting alone, it's also useful to do so with other people—especially those who understand what it takes to live a fit and healthy life. Talk to your family, friends, mentors, and anyone else who shares a similar mind. It's often the case that involving other people in your reflections will enable you to arrive at even more profound and useful realizations.

Commit to taking the time to reflect. Aim to unlock the specific ingredients that work for you best, and then latch on to them.

Final Word:

This book will right away assist you in moving your life onto a lean, optimized path. Much of what I've presented here will require time to absorb. Experiment with the various strategies and don't expect the impossible. Always remember that building the lean body should be regarded as a long-term effort—you'll need time to fully perfect your exercise, diet, and lean lifestyle. What I provide is a general approach that's useful for everyone, yet each individual's path towards attaining the lean body is a unique one. Adhere to the *The Lean Body Manual* as closely as possible, but tweak and adjust the program when necessary to fit your own path.

Congratulations! You're now ready to build the lean, athletic, V-12 body.

I wish you the best of luck.

THE 5 SECRETS
TO THE LEAN BODY

The 5 Secrets to the Lean Body

1. Go As Hard As You Can For Long As You Can

Focus on the intensity of the workout, not the length. You're better off exhausting your body in 20 minutes than going half-pace for two hours.

2. Make Your Workout a Ritual

Warm up before each and every workout with a disciplined routine, which should always include at least 10 minutes of running at a 70% pace. Follow through with a drawn-out stretching after your training. A warm-up before your workout and a thorough stretch after will allow you to avoid injury so you can get lean and stay lean for the long run.

3. The Proportion of the Portion

Eat a full meal at each sitdown and focus on the proportion of the portion. You should seek to construct a plate of roughly 50% carbs, 30% vegetables and healthy fat (avocado), and 20% protein. This will allow you to feel full for many hours after your meal, and you will have substantial energy to power through your day. Don't fall for carb-free regimens. Having a full meal will allow you to eat less overall, control portion size, and move on from eating once your meals have finished.

4. Start Your Day Light

Contrary to common belief in America, breakfast should be your smallest meal of the day (only 2-3 bites of a carb dense food, just so that you have something in your stomach). Burn off the calories from dinner to fuel your morning workout.

5. Get Hot

Work out in the warmest conditions possible. If you're working out in the gym, wear sweatpants and a sweatshirt. Consider your elevated body temperature to be a supplement to your training. Your body will be working harder and you will benefit from the highest possible intensity in your workout.

PART IV:
THE LEAN BODY FITNESS PROGRAM

THE LEAN BODY
WARM-UP

The Lean Body Warm-Up

A) Run

- Run for 10 minutes at 70% of your maximum speed. By the end of your run, your heart rate should be elevated and you should be perspiring.

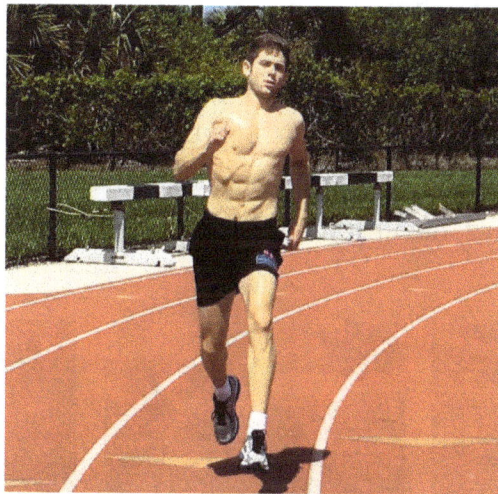

The following exercises (B through H) should be completed 2 times, 15 yards distance each time (find an open space and go back and forth for each exercise). For the Side Shuffle and Karaoke, be sure to complete each of the two repetitions moving towards a different side (once to your right and once to youe left).

B) Side Shuffle

- Position yourself in an athletic stance with your knees bent and your weight centered.

- Power sideways. As you move, you should elevate off the ground slightly and your feet should maintain distance from one another, never touching.

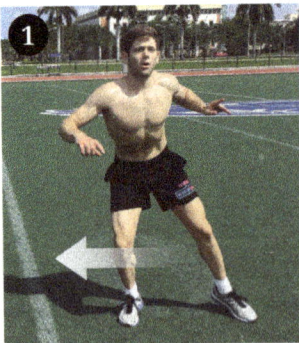

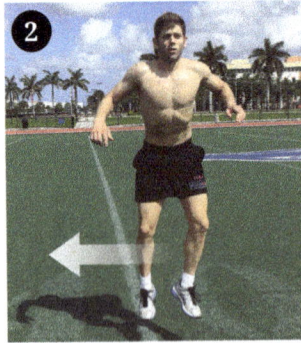

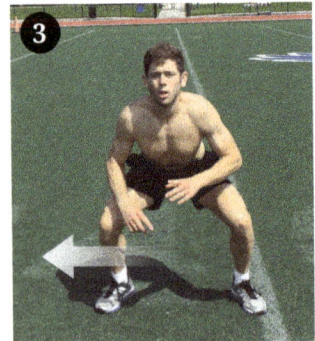

C) Karaoke

- Face forward with your feet shoulder length apart and your arms elevated, slightly below shoulder height.

- When moving to your right: cross your left foot over your right foot and rotate your torso in the same direction. Your left arm should move to the right (in coordination with the crossover step) and across your body and your right arm should move backwards (your arms should be like helicopter blades).

- As you make the next step sideways with your right foot, your arms should swing back into the neutral position.

- Your left foot now steps behind your right leg as your right arm moves across the front of your body and your left arm moves behind you. Again, your torso turns with the movement, but now in the opposite direction from where you're moving.

- It might take some time to perfect the coordination. Follow the above directions when moving to your left-hand side, but in the reverse.

- Remember: When stepping across the front of your body, the arm on the side of the crossing foot should move in that same direction. When your foot crosses behind your body, the arm on the opposite side of the crossing foot should move across your body.

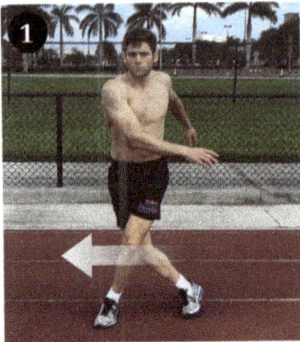
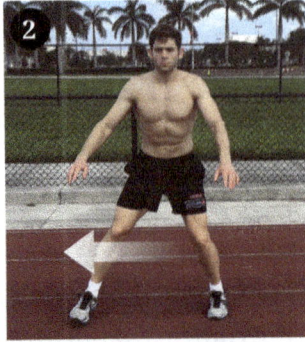
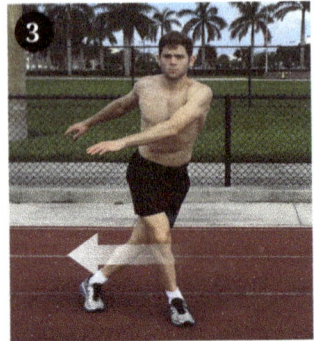
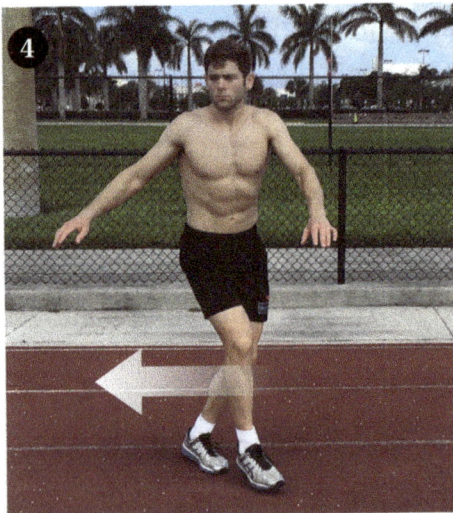
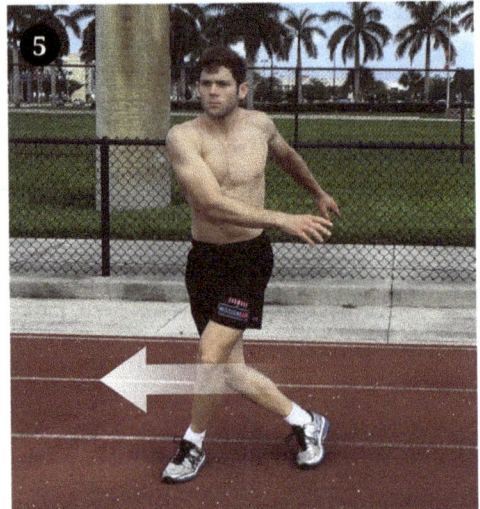

D) High Knees

- Move forward as you elevate each leg upwards.

- Your knee should reach at least navel height on each raise. Note: The focus should be on getting the knee up as high as possible, not on how much forward distance you cover with each step.

- Only one foot should be touching the ground at any given time, so you are transitioning directly from one leg raise to the next.

- Swing your arms in coordination with your steps as if you are running. Power your arm swings to raise your legs as high as possible

- Focus on keeping your back straight. Many people tilt their weight backwards in this exercise to accommodate the raise of the legs. Overcome this mistake by concentrating on shifting your center of gravity forward (while you may have the sensation that you're too far forward and hunched over, the end result is usually neutral).

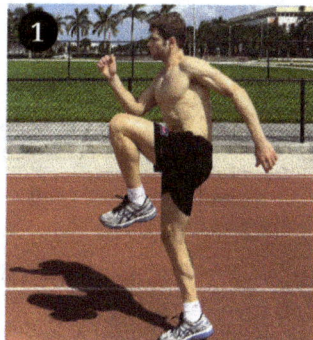

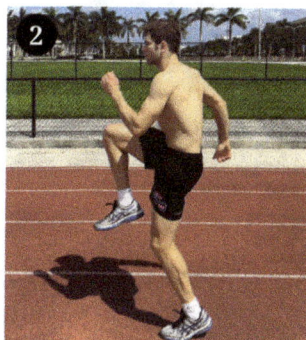

E) Butt Kicks

- Move forward as you bring your heel as close as possible to your butt.

- Like in the high knees exercise, only one foot should be touching the ground at any given time, so you are transitioning direclty from one kick to the next.

- One strategy for making the most of this drill is to put your hands behind your butt (palms facing backwards) and attempt to touch your heel to your palm. Feeling the foot on the hand with each rep will reaffirm that you're getting your leg up high enough.

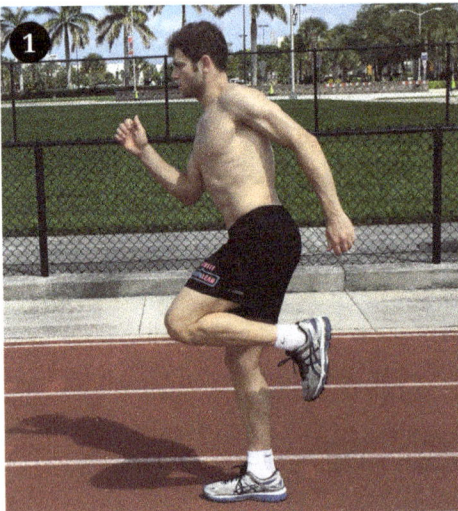

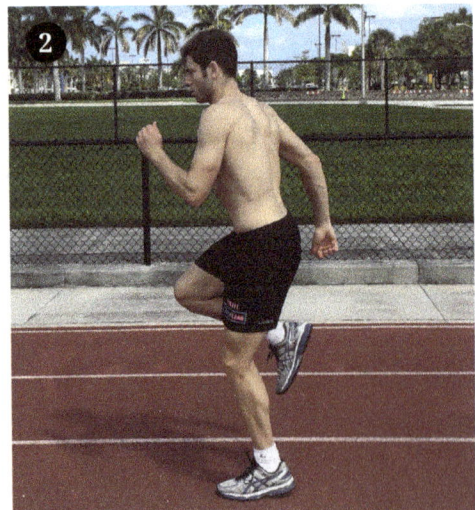

F) Arm Circles

- Skip forward as you circle both arms behind you, then over your head, and in front of you.

- Focus on syncing the rhythm of your skips to the movement of your arms.

- Try to get the widest possible arc with your arms. You want to feel your arms stretching and loosening in this drill, specifically in the shoulder blades, biceps, and bicep tendons.

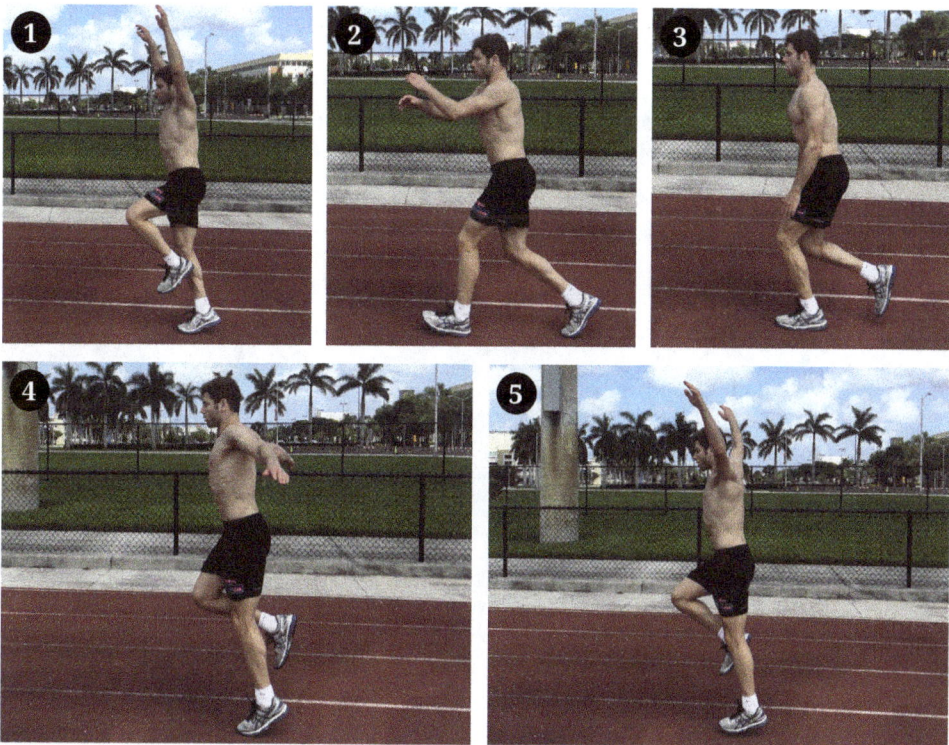

G) Arm Crosses

- Skip forward as you cross your arms in front of your body, and then open them up behind you.

- Focus on syncing the rhythm of your skips to the movement of your arms.

- Each time you bring your arms forward for the cross, alternate which arm goes above the other.

- You should feel your shoulders stretching with each cross, and you'll likely find that your arms move further and further behind you on the "open" segement of the drill.

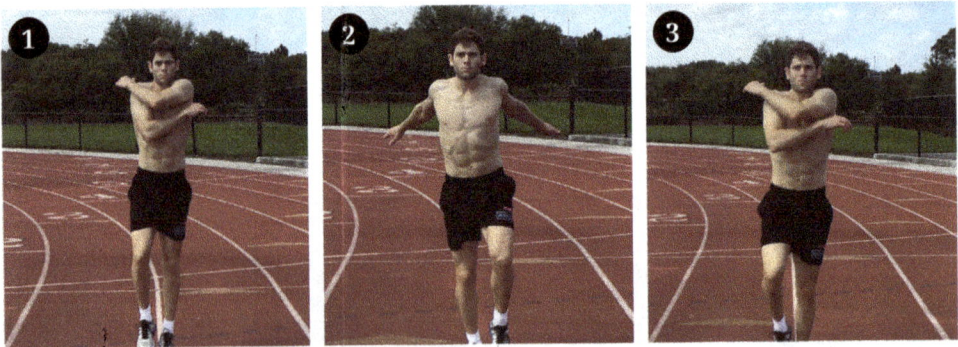

H) Power Skips

- Power yourself upwards with your knee raising alongside the opposite arm.

- Focus on the height of your jump as opposed to the forward distance covered with each step.

- After the skip, land on one foot (the leg that isn't raised) and then bring the foot of the raised leg to the ground too. For a brief moment, both legs will be touching the ground before you power up again with the opposite leg. The key is to have both feet on the ground at the same time for the least amount of time possible—you should immediately transition into the next skip.

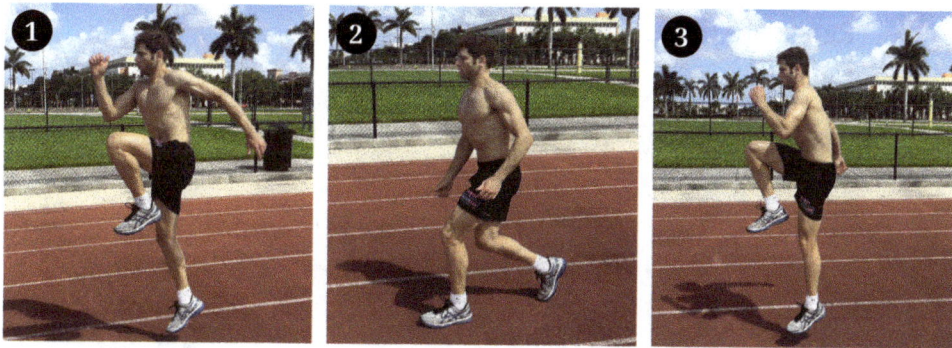

The following 3 exercises (I through K) are part of the Dynamic Stretching routine. Unlike the prior drills, these moves should be done slowly, holding each position for 2-3 seconds before moving on.

I) Worm with Push-up

- Stand straight with both feet together and reach down to touch your toes. Feel the stretch in your hamstrings.

- Inch yourself forward with your hands until your facing downward in the push-up starting position.

- Complete one push-up at a normal pace and then walk your feet forward until you are again bending straight down and touching your toes. Hold this hamstring stretch for 2-3 seconds before walking your hands forward again.

- Repeat 10 times.

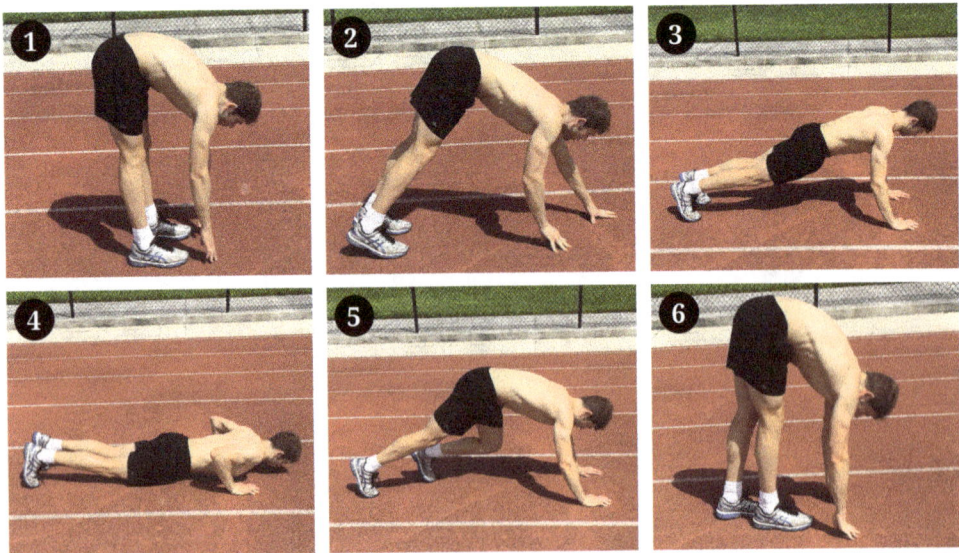

J) Spider with Hamstring Stretch

- Take a long step forward and bend the knee of your back leg so that it's hovering just above the ground.

- Support yourself with your hands on either side as you shift your body weight forward, until you feel the stretch in the hip flexor of your back leg.

- Use the arm on the side of your forward leg to stabilize yourself, pressing that elbow against the inner thigh of the forward leg. The hand opposite your forward leg should be touching the ground to support you. Hold for 2-3 seconds.

- From that position, use your hands on either side to shift your body weight backwards while straightening out your front leg. You should feel a strong stretch in the upper hamstring of the forward leg. Hold for 2-3 seconds.

- Step forward with your back leg and repeat on the opposite side. Complete 5 repetitions on each side.

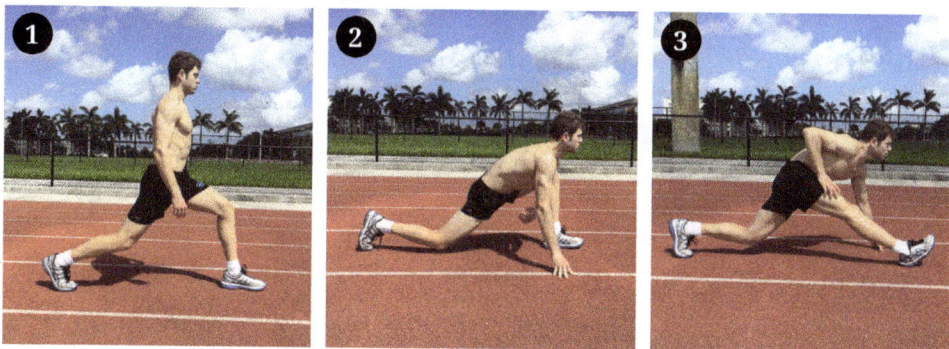

K) Quad Pulls

- Balance yourself on one leg while grabbing your other foot with the arm on the same side. Pull your heel to your butt and feel the stretch in your quadricep.

- Hold the stretch for 2-3 seconds before taking a step forward and repeating with the other leg. Complete 5 repetitions on each side.

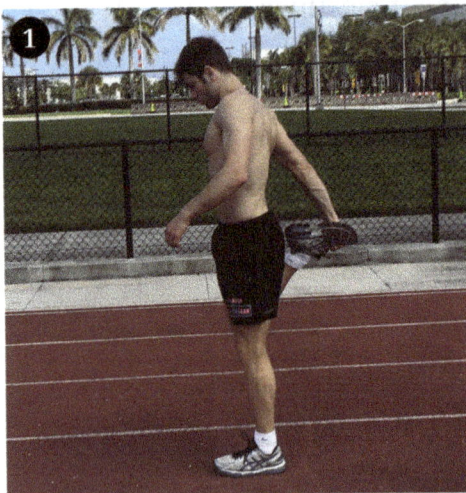

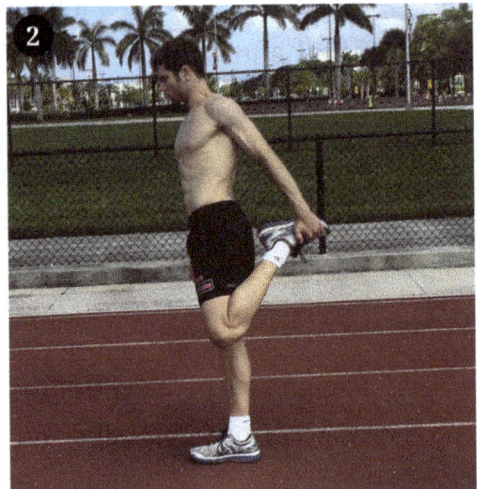

THE LEAN BODY
ARM AND CORE
WORKOUT

The Lean Body Arm and Core Workout

All of the exercises are explained in detail in this section. The number of repetitions will vary depending upon your current fitness level. Some exercises in this routine are grouped together, which means that they should be completed continuously, the only rest time being the few seconds it takes you to transition from one exercise to the next. You may have to complete several sets in the same grouping before moving on to the next exercise.

Exercises A through D represent the first group. You should complete the full circuit of these four exercises 3 times before moving on to exercise E.

A) Pull-Ups

- Grip the pull-up bar with your hands, which should be in line with your shoulders.

- With your arms extended, lift your chin to the height of the bar.

- Bring yourself back down until your arms are fully extended and repeat.

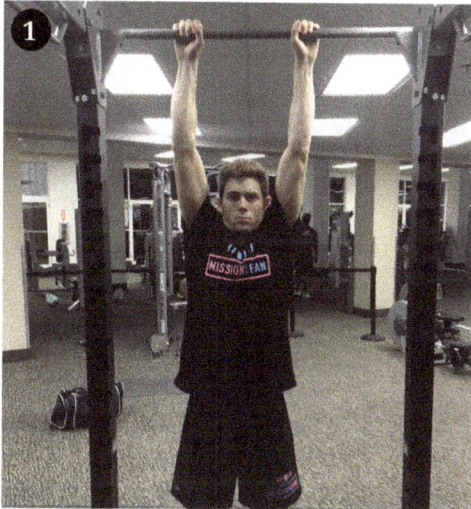

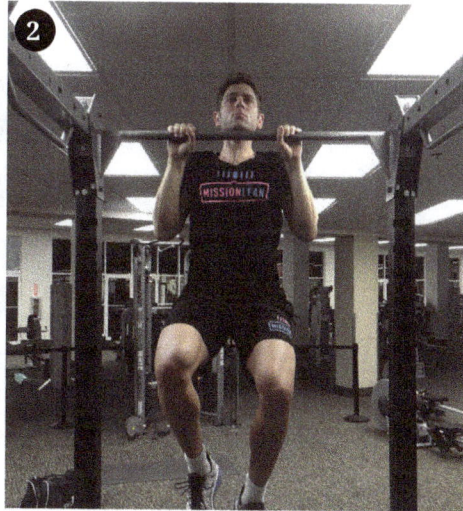

B) Push-Ups

- The traditional push-up.

- Keep your back straight and bring your body as low to the ground as possible. Bring yourself back up so that your arms are fully extended.

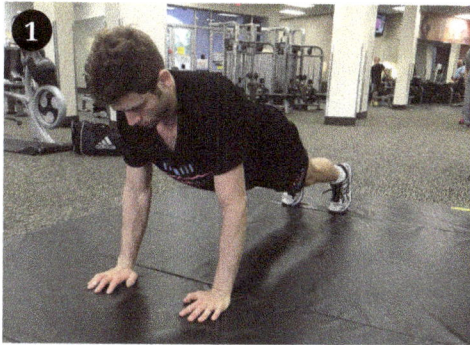

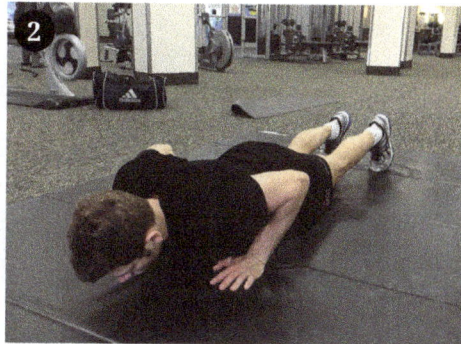

C) Sit-Ups

- Lay on your back with your hands behind your head and your feet above the ground in the crossed position.

- Raise your head, bringing your elbows as close to your knees as possible.

- Focus on using the contraction of your abdomen to lift yourself, not your neck. Also, focus on bringing your elbows up towards the sky as opposed to laterally, towards your feet.

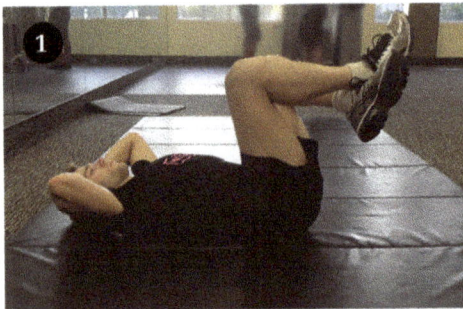

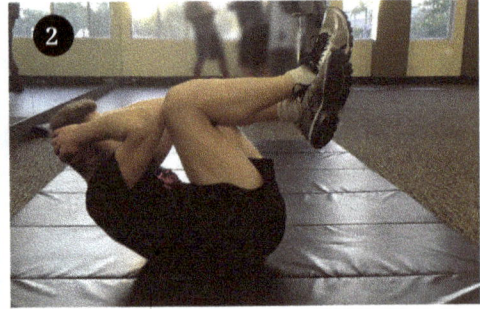

D) 45 Degree Back Extension

- Adjust the machine so that your hips are positioned roughly six inches above where the leg support ends.

- Cross your arms and allow your upper body to drop, still maintaining strength in your core.

- Lift yourself so that your body is *almost* completely aligned (not all the way, though, as you want to avoid hyperextending). Feel the move and what's comfortable for you in terms of how high you elevate. The most important part of this exercise is the initial movement from the downward position upwards, not the height of the raise. The muscles of your lower back should be working to elevate you.

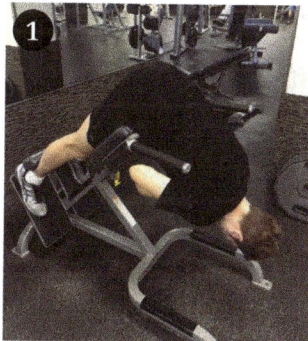

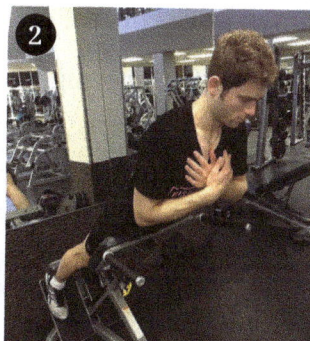

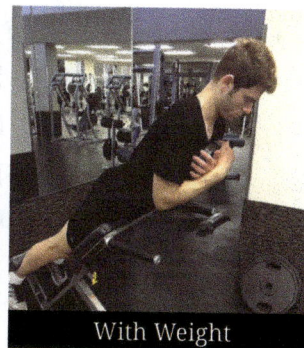

With Weight

Exercises E and F are a grouping. After finishing your set of military press, move directly into the reverse pull-ups with no rest in between. You will complete 5 sets of these two exercises before moving on to Exercise G.

E) Military Press

- Feel for the textured area of the bar (there are two gripping areas on either side) to find a balanced hand position.

- Make sure that the height of the bar position is comfortable (it's better to have it slightly lower than higher).

- Use your knees and core to assist you in taking the weight off the rack.

- Hold the bar at collar bone level and then extend the bar straight upwards. After your arms have fully extended, bring the weight back down with control to the original position.

- The goal should be to lift the weight with your arm strength alone, so limit the movement in your legs and feet (although you will still experience some movement regardless as part of the kinetic chain).

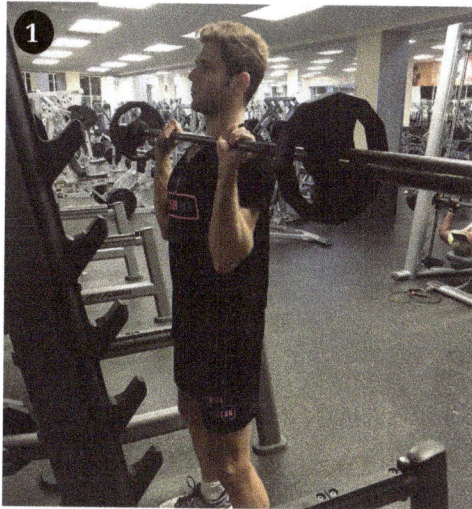

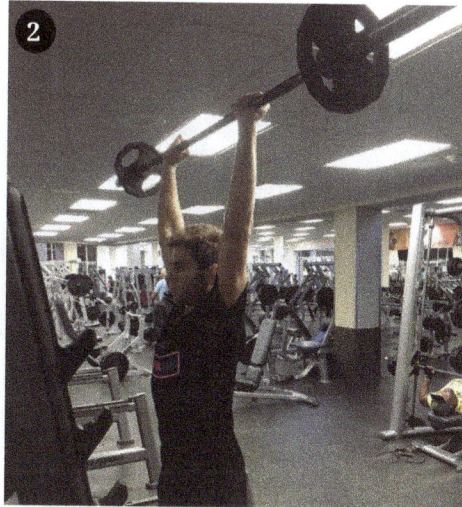

F) Reverse Pull-Ups

- Lay on the ground with the bar (I use a Smith machine) over you. The height of the bar should be such that keeping your arms straight will result in a position where you're elevated above the ground.

- Pull your body up until your chest touches the bar and then extend your arms as you descend.

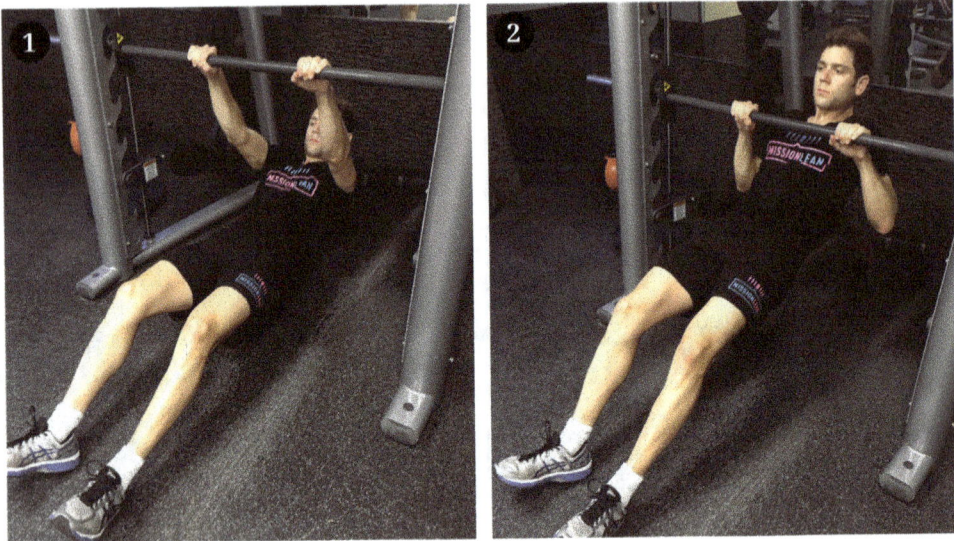

G) Deadlift

- Complete this exercise with your shoes off.

- Instead of picking the weight up off the floor to start this exercise, you can use a squat rack to hold the bar at knee level.

- Find a comfortable grip (shoulder length apart or slightly wider), lift the weight off the squat rack, and walk back one or two steps with the bar.

- Find your stance (again, about shoulder length) and allow your toes to point outwards slightly.

- Before bending down, make sure your grip is tight but allow your arms to relax. Your arms should be straight (not flexed at all) and the weight of the bar should be "hanging" to the floor from your loose arms (you want your legs—hamstrings and glutes—and back to move the weight).

- Keep your back straight and look forward (use the mirror to maintain eye contact, which will allow you to keep your back aligned).

- Allow the bar to move straight down, bending your knees as the bar grazes past the front of your kneecaps. Finish the motion about two-thirds of the way down your shin (if you're using 45 pound plates on either side, you should stop right at the point where the weights are about to touch the ground).

- Power up with your back and legs. Both the up and down movement should be controlled throughout.

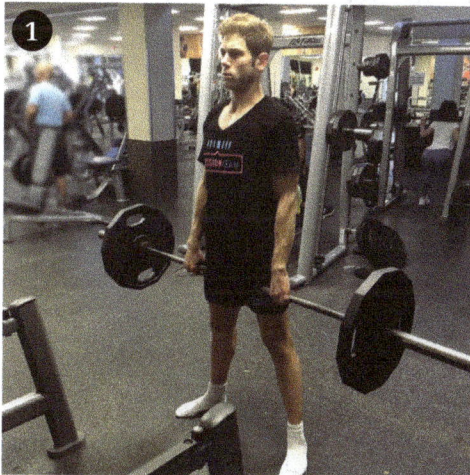

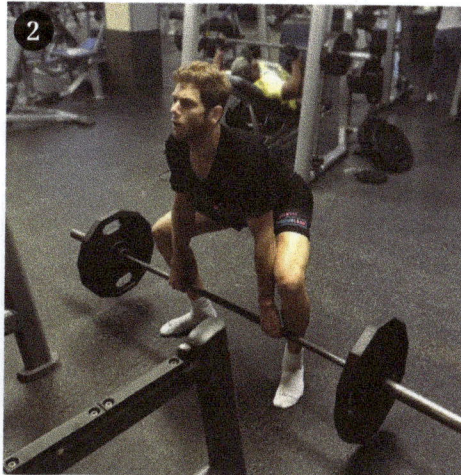

Exercises H and I should be done together. After finishing your set of bench press, move directly into the push-ups with no rest in between. You will complete 5 sets of these two exercises before moving on.

H) Bench Press

- Lay back on the bench with the bar positioned above you. The bar should be aligned with your chin while it's resting on the rack.

- Keep your feet on the ground and shuffle your shoulder blades inwards so that you can feel them touching bench.

- Find the textured area of the bar to find an even grip, and lift the bar up with full arm extension.

- In a controlled movement, bring the bar down to your chest and then straight up again, fully extending your arms.

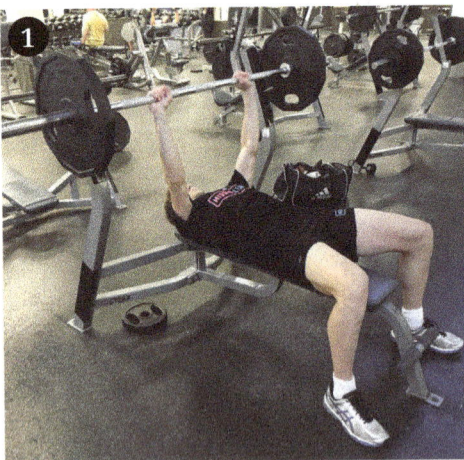

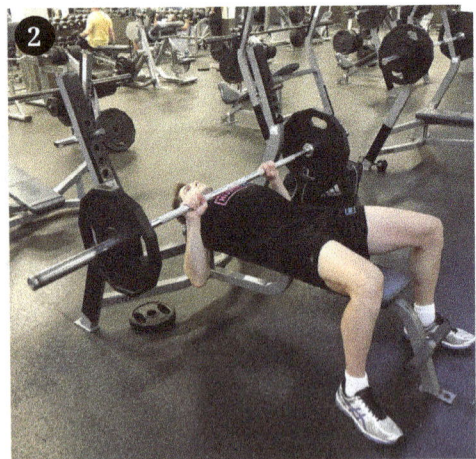

I) Push-Ups

- Immediately upon finishing your bench press set, move to the floor and complete a set of push-ups. The number of push-ups will be provided based upon your fitness level.

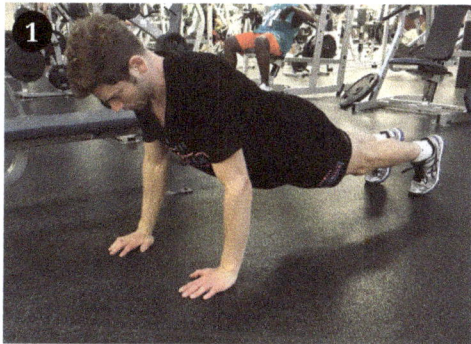

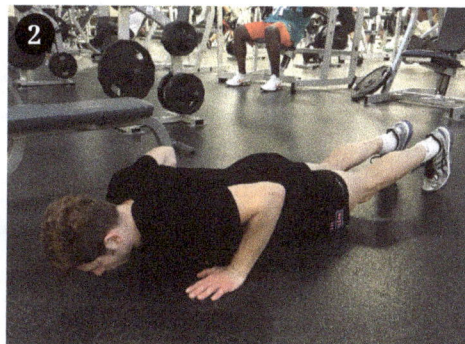

Exercises J and K should be done together. After finishing your set of Curl Press, move directly into the Arm Raises with no rest in between. You will complete 5 sets of these two exercises before moving on.

J) Curl Press

- Take two equal weight dumbbells in either hand.

- Curl your biceps, bringing the weight to shoulder level.

- Alter the wrist position slightly as you push the dumbbells up to the sky until your arms are fully extended.

- Bend your elbows, bringing the weight back to shoulder level and then drop your arms (make sure that when you bring the weight down from the upward extension, the point of change at the shoulder level is still included—as opposed to simply allowing the weight to drop down into a freefall).

- The motion should be fluid and continuous, and you should focus on the three points of the exercise (the weights at hip level, at shoulder level, and then fully extended upwards).

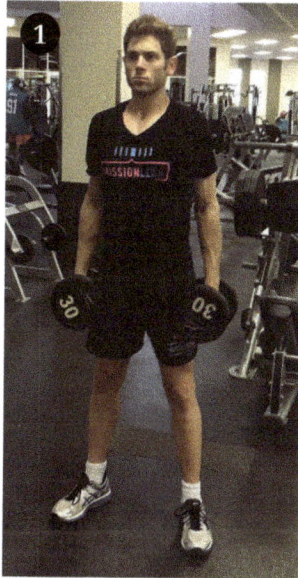

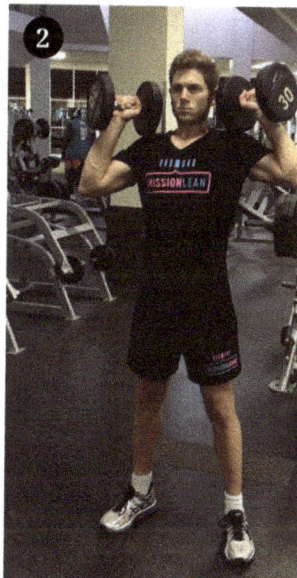

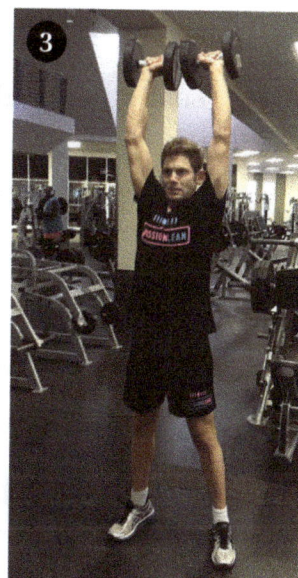

K) Arm Raises

- Hold equal weight plates in either hand with your arms by your side. Find a comfortable grip and use the center hole of the plate with your fingers as leverage.

- Look straight ahead. With your arms fully extended and your thumbs facing upward, lift the weights to just below shoulder height, and then back down again.

- The motion should be continuous and controlled, but done at a swift pace (a count of two to raise, and a count of two to lower).

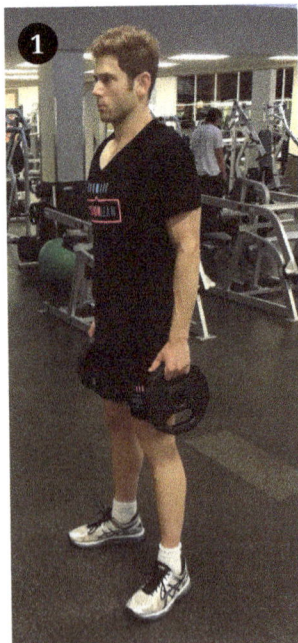

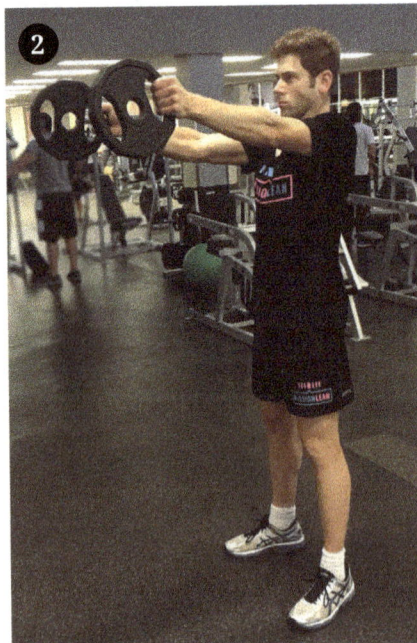

L) Rows

- Grab the grip with both hands and keep your back straight. The position should be such that with your arms are fully extended, the cables attached to the weight are firm (so that a slight pull will right away elevate the weight).

- Focus on bringing the shoulder blades together as you pull the cable to your chest. Look straight ahead and engage your core muscles.

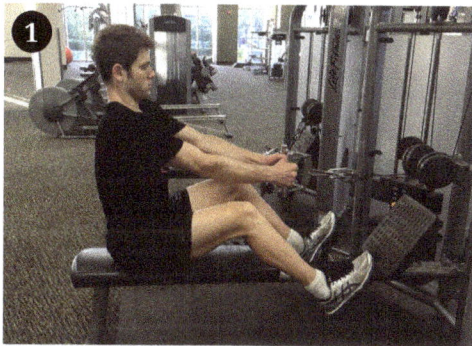

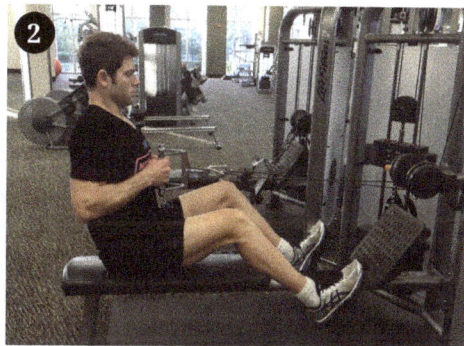

Exercises M and N should be done together. Move from one exercise to the next without rest (you will complete both variations in a row on one hand, before moving to the other hand). You will complete 5 sets of these two wrist exercises on each hand. The number of reps will vary depending upon your fitness level.

M) Wrist Raise

- Sit on a bench with your forearm resting on your knee and palm facing down holding the weight. Allow your wrist to bend downwards.

- Raise the weight straight up using your wrist. Keep your forearm and elbow in the same position in order to isolate your wrist.

- The motion should be controlled and fluid, both coming up and down. Complete with both wrists.

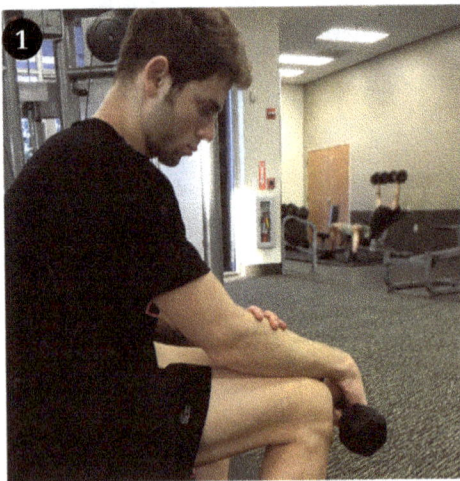

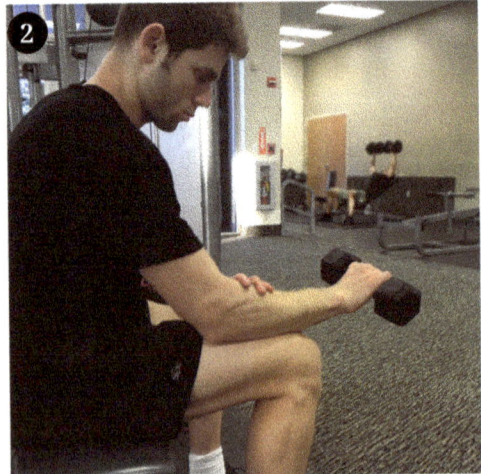

N) Wrist Curl

- Sit on a bench with your forearm resting on your knee and palm facing upwards while holding the weight. Allow the weight to roll down your palm and into your fingers.

- Move the weight with control from your fingers, to your palms, and then towards you as you curl your wrist.

- Once curled, move the weight slowly back down towards your fingers, allowing your palm to open and wrist to bend.

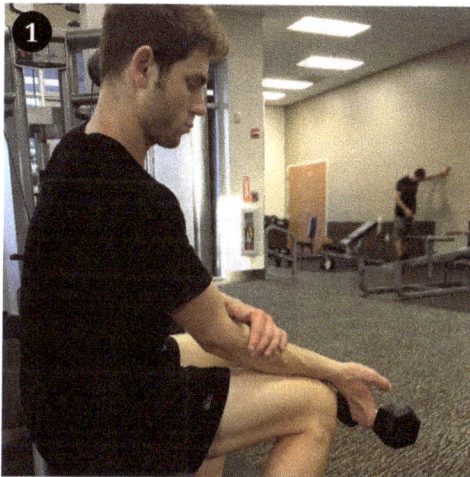

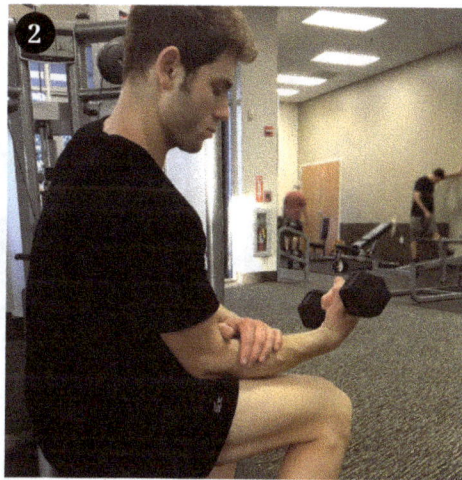

THE LEAN BODY LEG AND CORE WORKOUT

The Lean Body Leg and Core Workout

All of the exercises are explained in detail in this section. The number of repetitions will vary depending upon your current fitness level. Some exercises in this routine are grouped together, which means that they should be completed continuously, the only rest time being the few seconds it takes you to transition from one exercise to the next. You will need to complete several sets of the same grouping before moving on to the next exercise.

Exercises A and B are the first grouping, and should be done continuously. Right after you finish your set of squats, step back and immediately begin the squat jumps. You will complete several sets of these two exercises before moving on.

A) Squats

- Complete this exercise with your shoes off.

- Make sure that the bar height on the rack is comfortable (it's better to have the bar slightly lower than higher). Ideally, the bar should be about chest level on the rack.

- Step underneath the bar and allow the bar to rest on your trapezius muscles (while the bar may come into contact slightly with your center back and spine, the majority of the weight should be supported by your traps).

- Feel for the textured area of the bar (there are two gripping areas on either side) to find a balanced hand position.

- Bend your legs and then raise yourself into the upright position as the bar lifts off the rack. Step back one or two steps, and find your balance.

- Get into a comfortable stance (a bit wider than shoulder width is ideal) and allow your toes to point outwards slightly.

- Focus on keeping your back straight as you bend down into the squat position (make eye contact with yourself in the mirror as you do your squats—this will help keep your back straight).

- You should aim to squat down as far as you can. The ideal squat position is just before your knees reach a 90 degree bend (roughly a 100-110 degree angle).

- Complete your reps, stand upright, and then walk the weight forward until the bar hits both side beams of the rack. Only after the bar has made contact with the beams do you then bend down and place the weight on the hooks. This will allow you to avoid hurting yourself/missing the weight hooks when re-racking the bar.

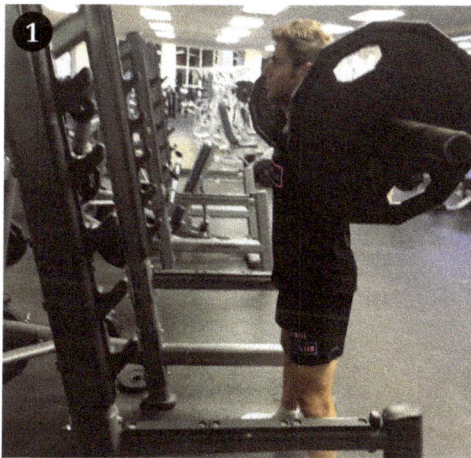

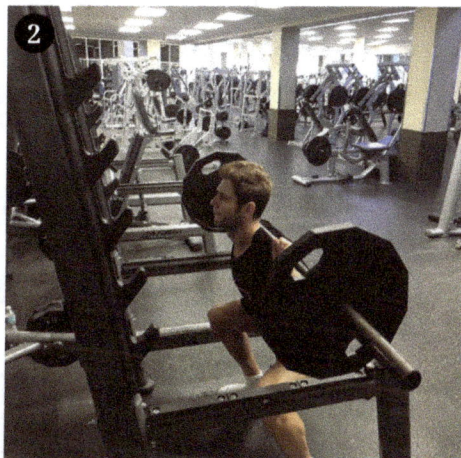

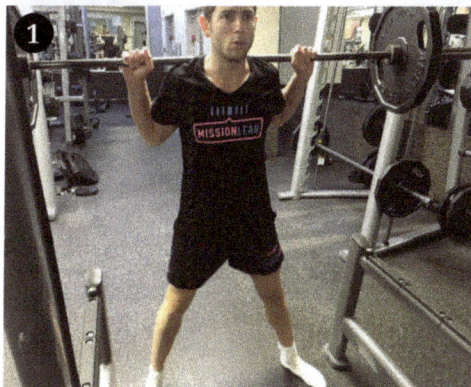

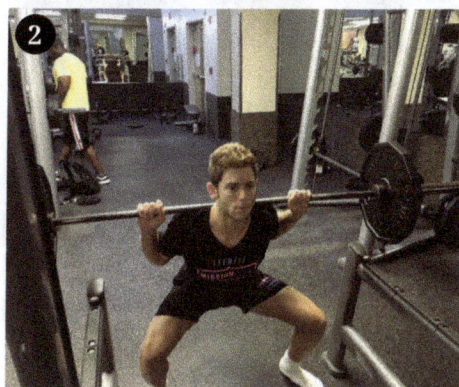

Two angles of this exercise (side and front) are pictured here.

B) Squat Jumps

- Position yourself in a bodyweight squat with your arms close to your legs, your back straight, and the burn of holding the position concentrated in your quads.

- Spring upwards as high as you can and reach your arms straight up towards the sky.

- When you land, focus on bending your knees as opposed to your back.

- The motion should be fluid, and you should immediately spring back upwards the moment you reach your final squatting position. There is no pause between jumps in the squatting position.

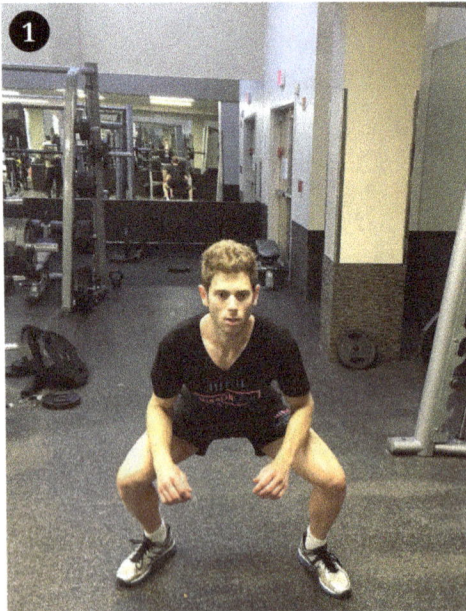

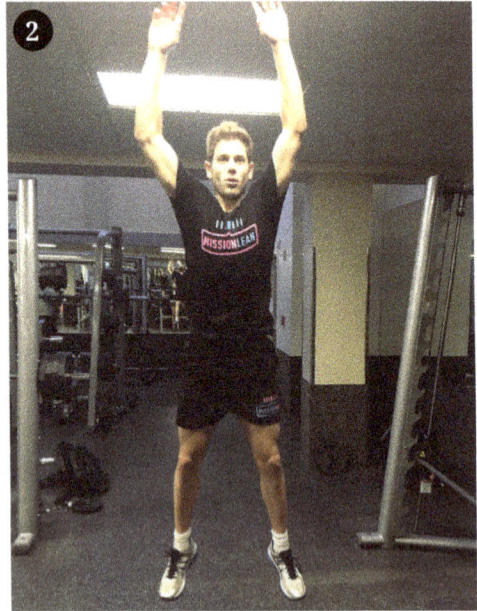

Exercises C and D are a grouping and should be done continuously. Right after you finish your set of lunges, step back and immediately begin the lunge jumps. You will complete several sets of these two exercises before moving on.

C) Lunges

- The bar height on the rack should be the same as you had for squats (about chest level).

- Step underneath the bar and allow the bar to rest on your traps.

- Feel for the textured area of the bar to find a balanced hand position.

- Move into the upright position as you lift the bar off the rack, step back three or four steps, and find your balance. Your legs should be straight and feet close together.

- Take a long step forward (about 70-80% of your full range) with one leg and bend your knee 90 degrees into the lunge position.

- Right away power back up and bring yourself to the standing position again. Repeat your full series of reps *on the same leg* before you move to the other leg.

- After you complete both sets on either leg, find your balance in the standing position and then walk the weight forward until the bar hits both side beams of the rack. Only after the bar has made contact with the beams do you slowly bend down until the bar finds the hooks. This will allow you to avoid hurting yourself/missing the weight hooks when re-racking the bar.

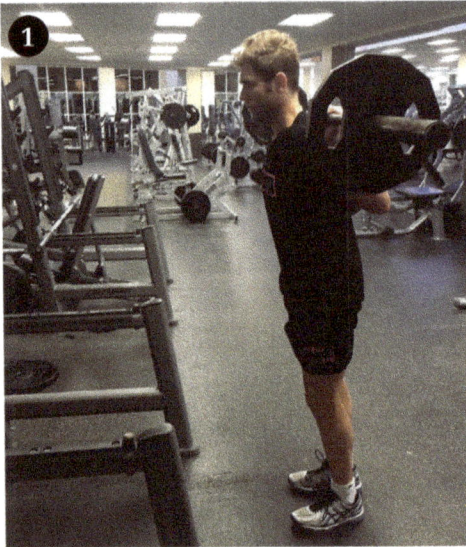

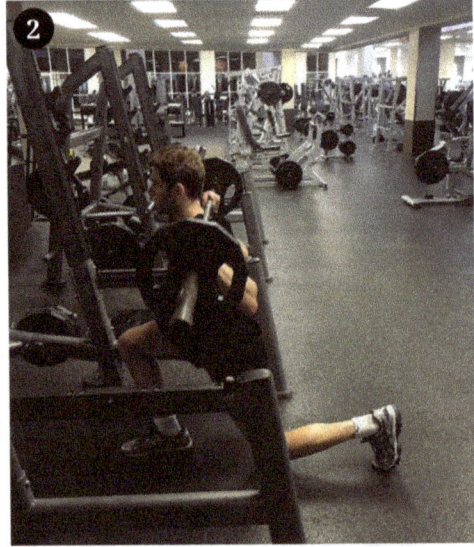

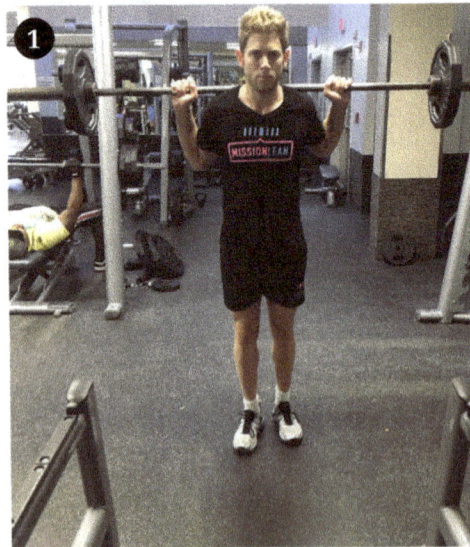

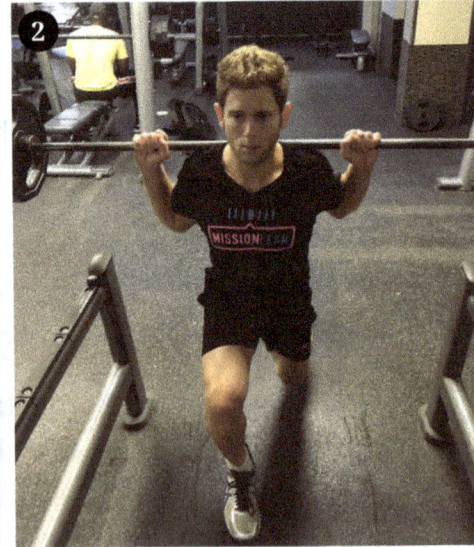

Two angles of this exercise (side and front) are pictured here.

D) Lunge Jumps

- Take a step forward and allow your back leg to bend, the knee hovering just above the ground.

- Spring upwards and alternate your legs in mid-air so that your back leg is now in front of you, and your front leg is behind you.

- Land in the same position (with your legs now reversed) and focus on bringing your back leg as close to the ground as possible.

- The motion should be fluid, and you should immediately spring upwards again the moment you reach your final lunging position. There should be no pause in the downward lunge position between jumps.

- Concentrate on jumping as high as you can.

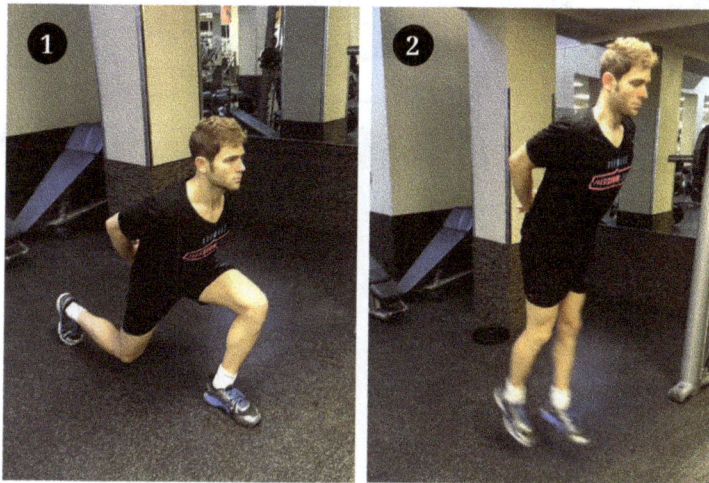

Exercises E, F, and G are a grouping and should be done continuously. Right after you finish one exercise, immediately move into the next. You will complete several sets of these three exercises before moving on.

E) Plank

- Bring your fists together and hold yourself in the plank position with your forearms and toes touching the ground.

- Focus on keeping your back straight, your body parallel to the ground.

- Allow the muscles of your core (abs and back) to support your weight.

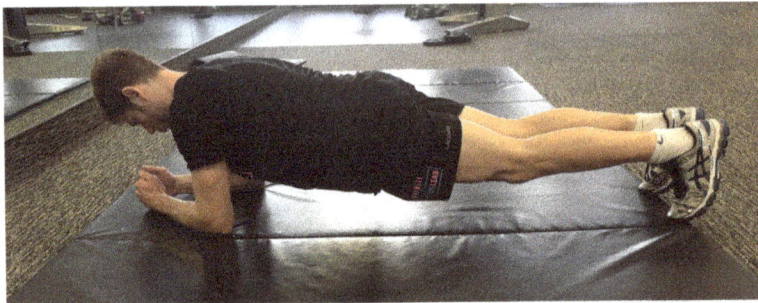

F) Superman

- Lay flat on your stomach with your arms fully extended in front of you. Lift your legs and arms up off the ground (not too high, about 6 inches).

- Focus on keeping your arms straight ahead of you (don't allow them to drift sideways).

- Look down and keep your neck straight.

- You should feel the muscles of your lower back working to support you. You will also feel your shoulders working to prevent your arms from drifting to the side.

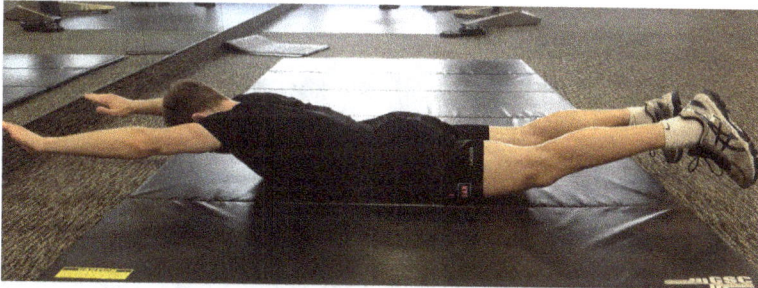

G) Bicycles

- Lay on your back on the matt, put your hands behind your head and lift your feet off of the ground.

- Bend one leg while keeping the other straight. As you bend your leg, bring the opposite elbow forward and try to touch your elbow to your knee.

- Reverse the movement now, straightening the bent leg and bending your other leg. Elevate the opposite elbow forward, bringing it as close to the knee as possible.

- This exercise should be done fluidly and continuously.

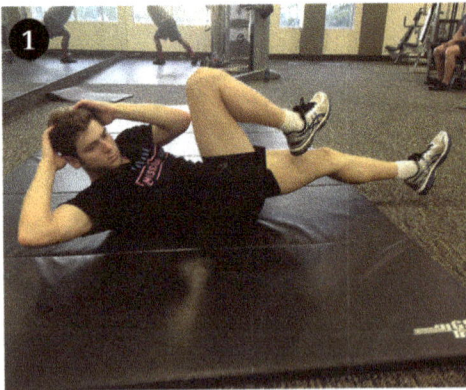

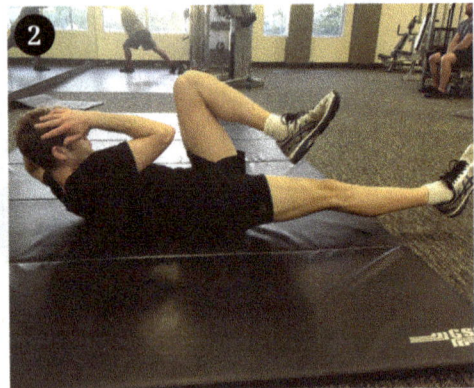

H) Leg Raises on Machine

- Adjust the backseat of the machine so that your knees are positioned right at the front ledge of the seat cushion. Adjust the angle of the machine's "arm" (the piece that elevates with your leg extension) so that your legs are bent underneath you at an angle slightly less than 90 degrees.

- Brace your core and lift your legs upwards until they are fully extended. You should feel your quadriceps muscles working here.

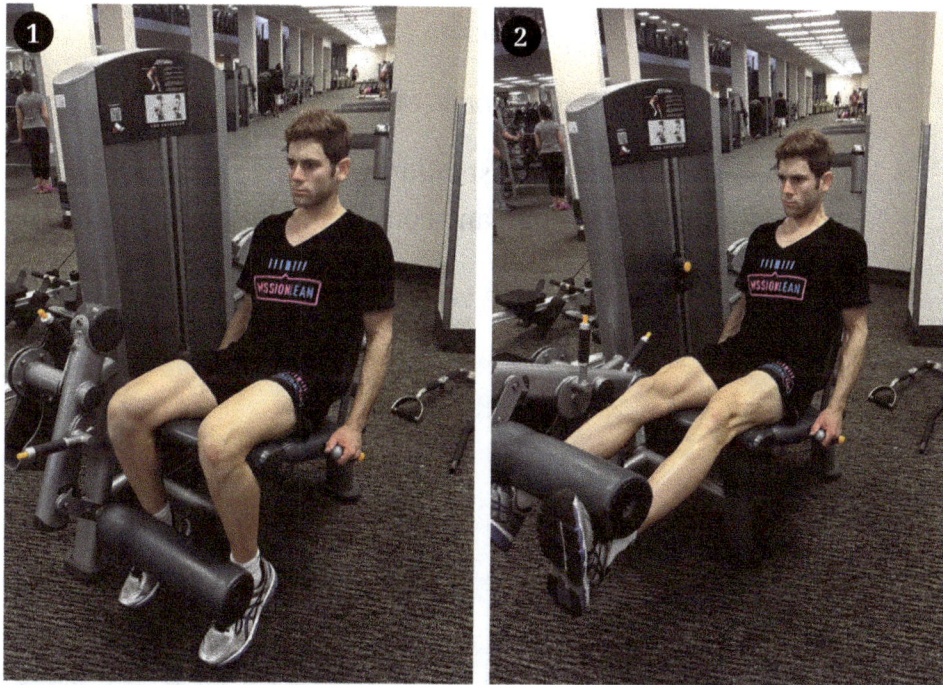

I) Swiss Ball Hamstrings

- Lay on your back, your heels positioned at the center of the Swiss Ball and your butt off the ground (and body completely straight). Keep your core firm, legs straight, and arms by your sides or on your chest. (There are various sizes of Swiss Balls—the right size ball should position your body at roughly a 20 degree angle from the ground when your body is completely straight.)

- Dig your heels into the Swiss Ball as you bend your knees and the ball rolls towards your butt. Get as much knee bend as possible, and allow your back to elevate off the ground.

- Straighten your legs as the ball returns to its original position.

- Your hamstrings and butt should be working in this exercise. The motion should be fluid and continuous as you move the ball back and forth.

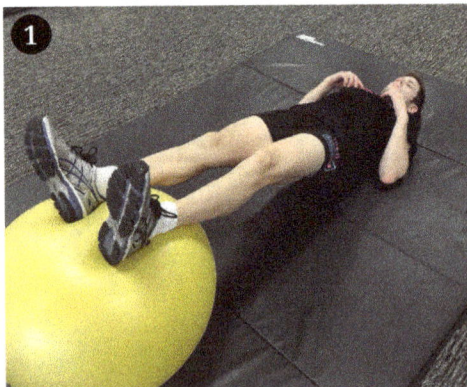

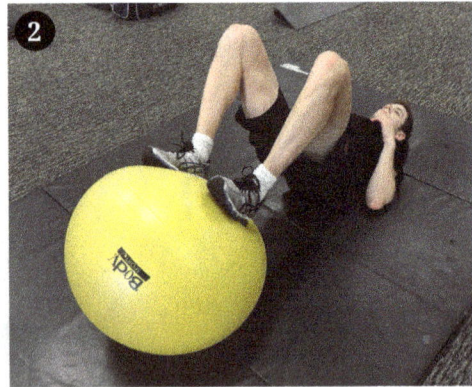

J) Calf Raises

- Find an optimal position on the machine where your legs are straight and your shoulders are in contact with the pads (you should feel the resistance of the weight pressing on your shoulders). Keep your heels pointed to the ground and your forefoot on the "step" of the machine. Hold the machine's grips if it has them.

- Elevate onto your toes as your heels raise. Feel your calves working.

- The exercise should be controlled and the movement continuous. Try to get as much range of motion as possible.

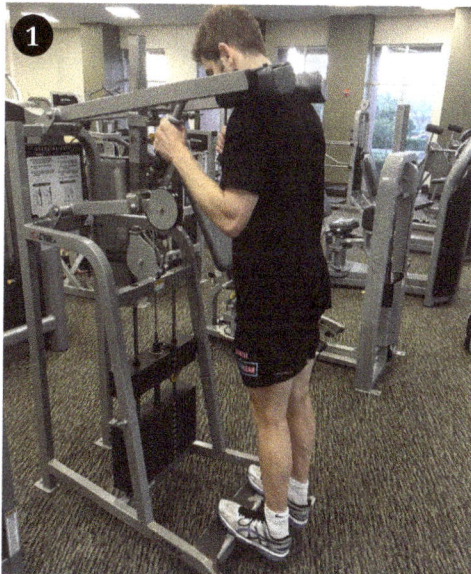

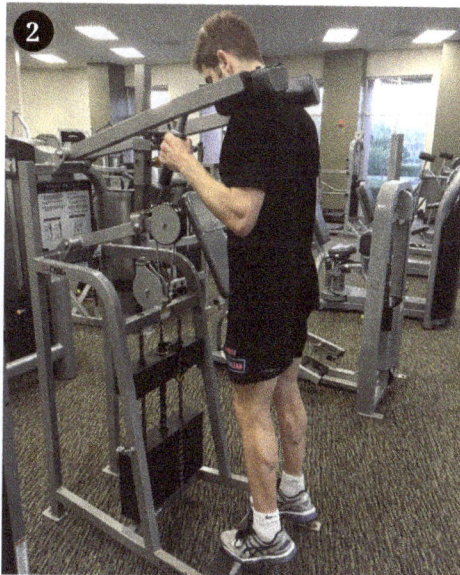

THE LEAN BODY
STRETCHING
ROUTINE

The Lean Body Stretching Routine

The Lean Body Stretching Routine should be done *after* your workout, when you are warm and limber. This routine is comprised of static stretches, each of which should be held for at least 10 seconds (stay in the position longer if you feel you need more). Be sure to focus on your breath during the stretches, using every exhale to move further into the position and find greater range of motion. The stretches are presented in the order they should be performed. You may implement some of these static stretches before your workout too, as a complement to the 3 *dynamic* stretching exercises in the Lean Body Warm-Up (if you do use the static stretches presented here *before* your workout, hold for around 5 seconds—holding static stretches for longer before a workout will hamper your performance in the training). I have included photos of the same stretch being done in various settings. This is to show that the routine can be completed virtually anywhere (the tennis court, the gym, the field, etc.). On off days, try to spend 15 minutes going through these stretches so you recover fully and are loose for the week's training program.

A) Glutes and Hips

- Raise your foot and lay it sideways on the bar/net/platform, at about hip level (grab your foot with your hand on the same side to assist you in raising the leg). The outside, middle portion of your foot should be resting on the surface. (Notice that when doing this stretch on the net, my raised foot is positioned at the higher point of the net—towards the net post—and my knee is stationed where the net is lower. Complete the stretch in this way if you have access to a tennis net. If you're doing this stretch on a straight bar or surface, don't worry about this point.)

- Lean forward above the elevated leg. Feel the stretch in your butt and hip. Adjust your body until you find the optimal position.

- If you're a beginner, you may complete this stretch by elevating your foot to a lower height. If you're using a tennis net, simply move your body more towards the center net strap, or if you're using a bar (a Smith Machine or other), adjust accordingly.

- If you benefit from advanced flexibility, try to bring your head to your knee. You may even be able to complete the stretch with your foot higher than the level of the tennis net (use a Smith Machine and raise the bar as high as you can manage). You will definitely need to use your hand to raise your foot to that level (use the hand on the same side of the leg you're raising—the opposite hand should be holding the bar for support).

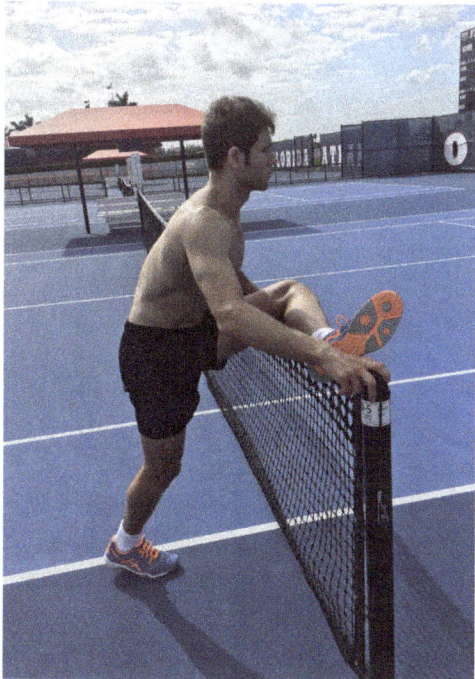
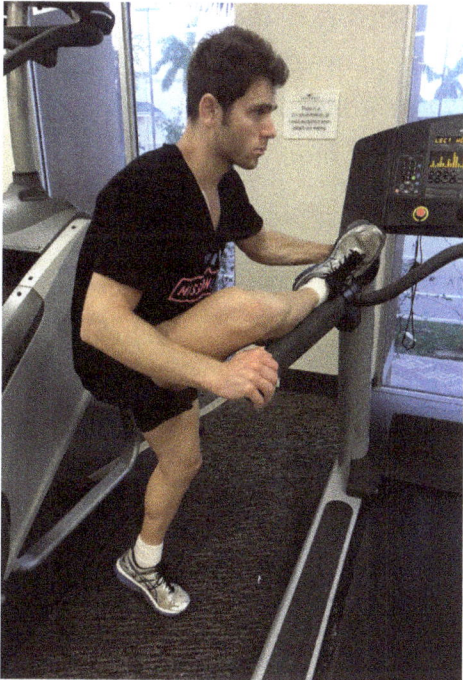

Stretches B through D should all be done in a row, with the leg kept elevated as you adjust from one stretch to the next. These three stretches can be done on the tennis net, the bar of a Smith Machine, or even on the treadmill handle bars.

B) Standing Hamstring

- Lift up your foot onto the bar/net/platform at about hip level. Your heel should be resting on the surface with your toes pointing up.

- Face forward and lean in. Keep your back straight and reach for your toes (touch them if you can).

- Keep your foot elevated when you're finished with this stretch because you will be transitioning directly into the next stretch, the Standing Groin.

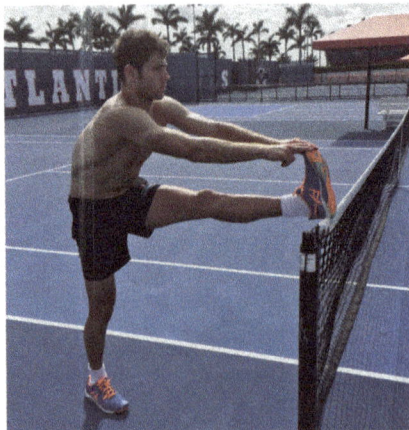

C) Standing Groin

- With your foot still elevated from the Standing Hamstring stretch, rotate the foot that's on the ground so that your body turns 90 degrees and you're in an open stance.

- Lean forward and away from your elevated foot so that you feel the stretch in the groin on the elevated leg.

- For those who are advanced, you will again want to transition directly into the next stretch—the Quad Stretch—without bringing down the elevated foot.

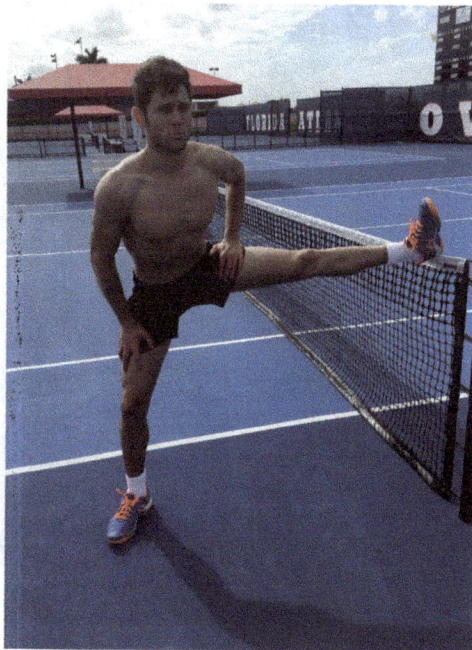

D) Quad Stretch

- If you're transitioning into this stretch directly from the Standing Groin stretch, simultaneously flip your foot over (so the top is resting on the bar/net/surface) and inch your body back (toward the elevated leg) with the foot that's on the ground.

- Once in the correct position, adjust yourself (you may need to lean back or bend the leg that's on the ground slightly) until you feel a solid stretch in the quadricep of the elevated leg.

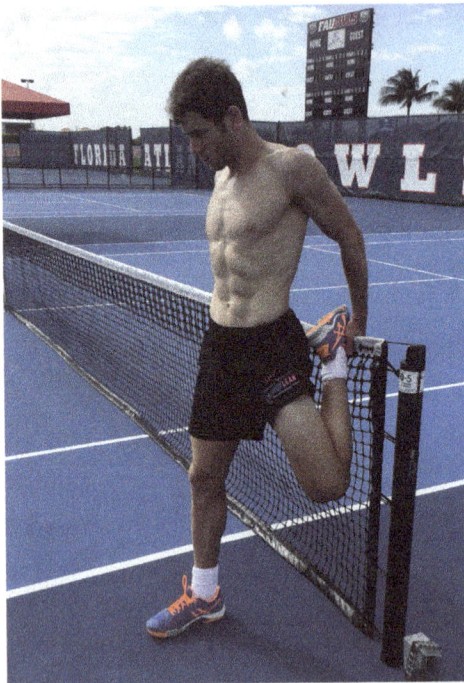

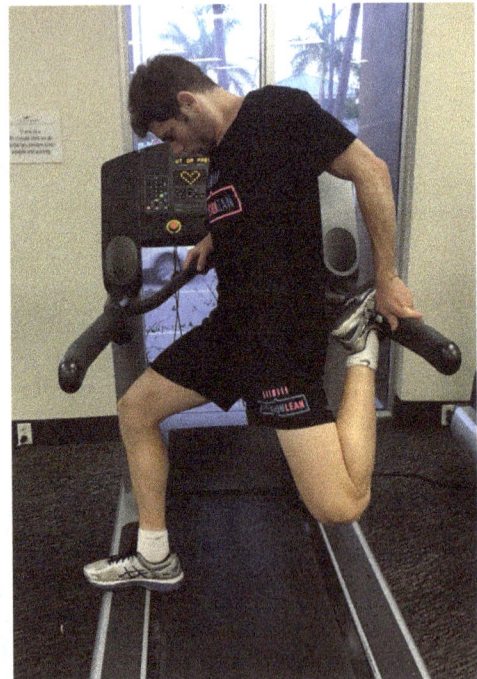

E) Arm Pull

- Again, use a tennis net or a bar/surface that's hip level or higher, and hold with both hands shoulder width (or slightly wider) apart.

- With an athletic stance, bring your butt backwards and bend your knees so that your arms are straight and your head is facing down.

- You should feel this stretch in your shoulders, upper back, neck, and bicep tendons.

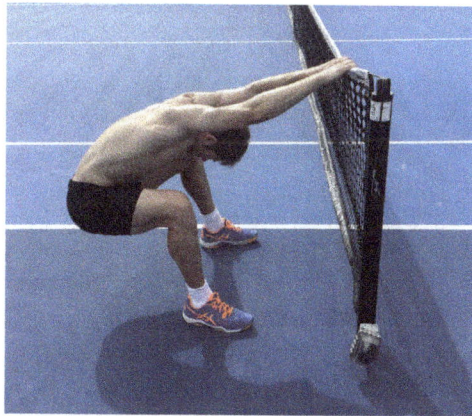

F) Butterfly

- Stand with your back to the net/bar and grab the surface with both hands behind you (try to get them as close together as you feel comfortable), so that your arms are fully extended.

- Lean your chest forward and allow your head to bend back slightly.

- You should feel this stretch in your shoulders, biceps, and bicep tendons. You may adjust your position to feel the stretch more in one shoulder or the other. Gauge your feelings to find the right pose.

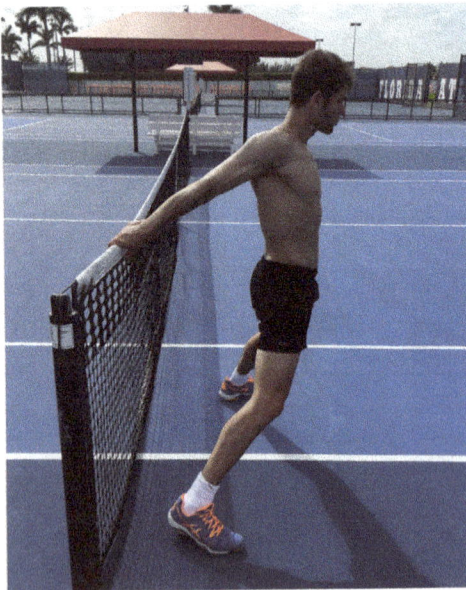

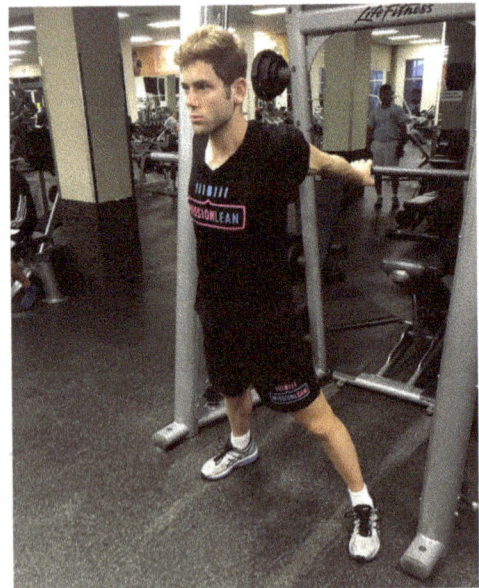

Stretches G and H should be done together, so after you've completed the hamstring stretch (G) and returned to the upright sitting position, move directly and fluidly into the lower back stretch (H). These two stretches are great complements to one another, and they will allow you to get the most range of motion when done together.

G) Sitting Hamstring

- Sit on the floor with your legs extended out in front of you, feet touching.

- Reach for your toes (touch them if you can), extending your arms forward. Lean into the stretch and breathe.

- As you release and move backwards, move directly into the next stretch (lower back), "H."

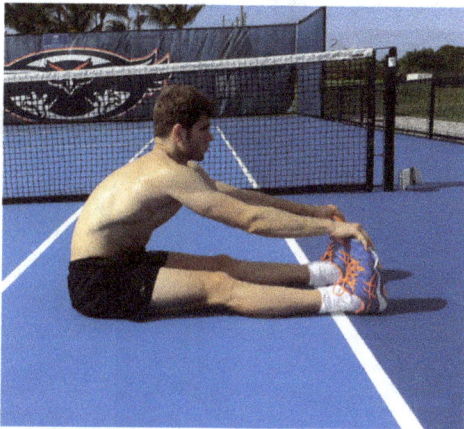

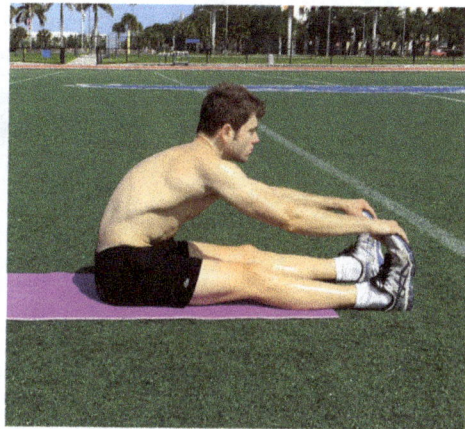

H) Lower Back: Feet Over Your Head

- Lay flat on your back with your arms straight above your head and back of the hands touching the ground.

- Use your abs to lift your legs straight up and over your head, grabbing your toes with your palms.

- If you aren't flexible enough yet in the beginning, simply bring your feet as far over your head as possible until you feel the stretch in your lower back (the third picture shows a halfway pose).

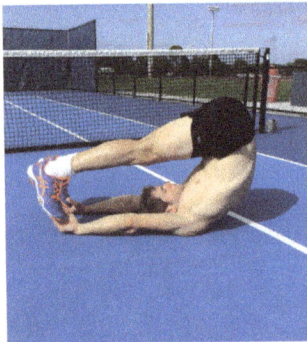

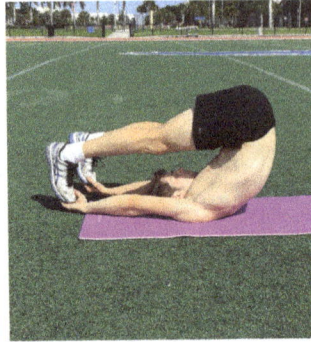

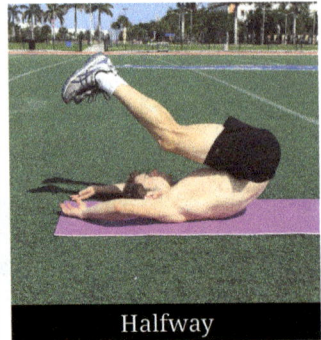

Halfway

I) Sitting Groin

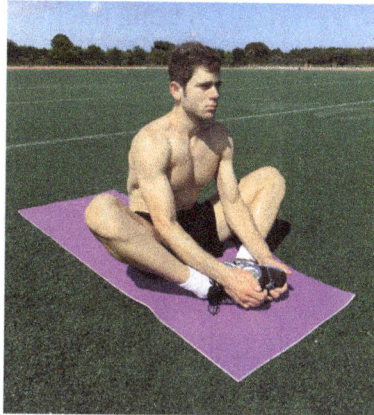

- Sit on your butt and bring the bottoms of your feet together.

- Hold your feet with your hands and lean your weight forward until you feel the stretch on both sides of your groin.

- As you get more flexible, try to bring your head as close as possible to your feet.

J) Sitting Glute

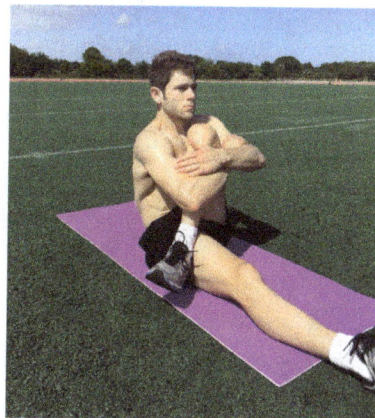

- Sit on the ground with both legs extended.

- Cross one leg over the other and wrap both arms around the crossed leg, hugging it close to your chest.

- Feel the stretch in the glute of the crossed leg.

K) Laying Down: Hip and Glute

- Lay on your back and lift your knees up off the ground, keeping them bent.

- Cross one leg over the other so that the outside ankle of the crossed leg rests on the lower quadricep (just before the bend of the knee) of the other.

- Interlock your hands *behind* your knee (inside the crevice of the bend) and pull your leg towards you. It's important that your hands pull from inside the crevice, and *not* from outside (on the shin), as this would put a strain on the knee.

- You should feel the stretch in the hip and glute of the crossed leg.

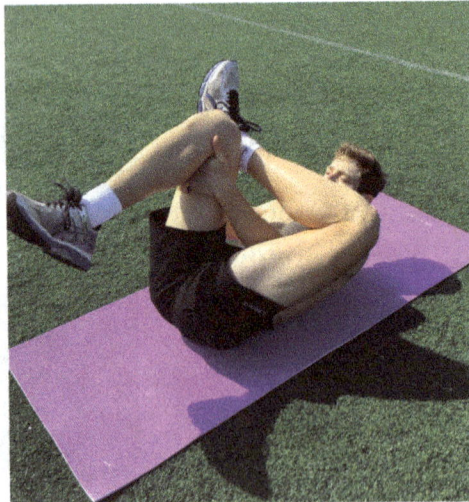

L) Hip Flexor

- Position yourself in a lunge position, with your back knee touching the ground lightly.

- If you have access to a tennis net or some other support, use it to assist you in this stretch. Otherwise, you may complete the stretch free-standing with your hands on your hips, or touching your fingertips to the ground on either side for support.

- Lean your bodyweight forward until you feel the stretch of the hip on the back leg.

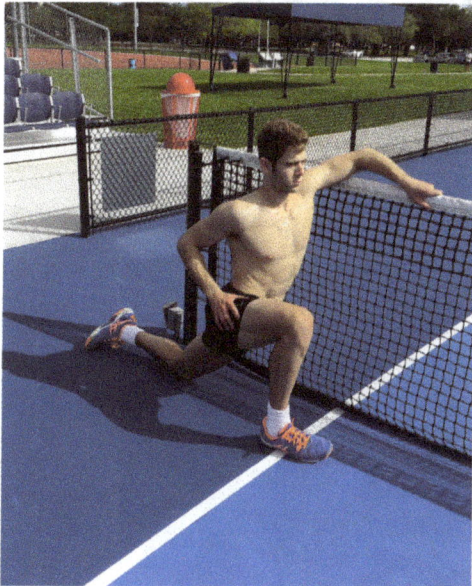

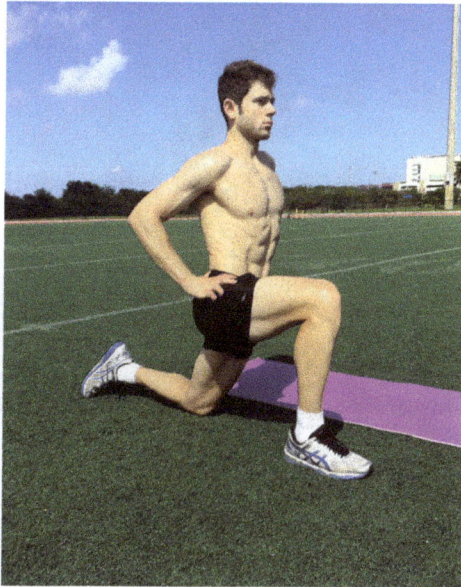

M) Calf Bend

- Position yourself as close to the wall as possible and bend your foot. Your foot should be angled so that your forefoot is touching the wall and your heel is against the ground.

- Move your weight in towards the wall until you feel your calf stretching in your forward leg.

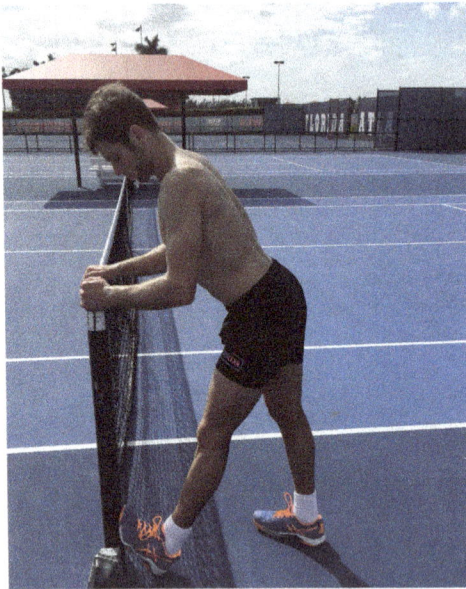

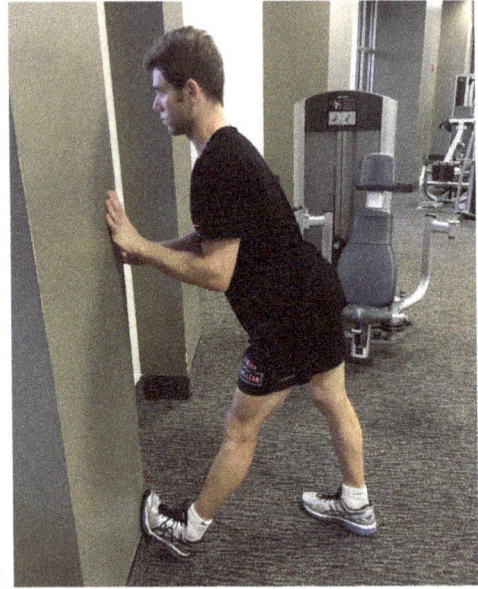

N) Calf Wall Push

- Put both hands on the wall and one leg in front of the other at a comfortable distance.

- Slant your hips forward so that your front knee bends and the heel of your back leg comes up off the ground.

- Push with your arms against the wall and use the force to bring the heel of the back leg onto the ground.

- You should feel the achilles and calf stretching on the back leg.

- This stretch should be done barefoot to maximize the range of motion.

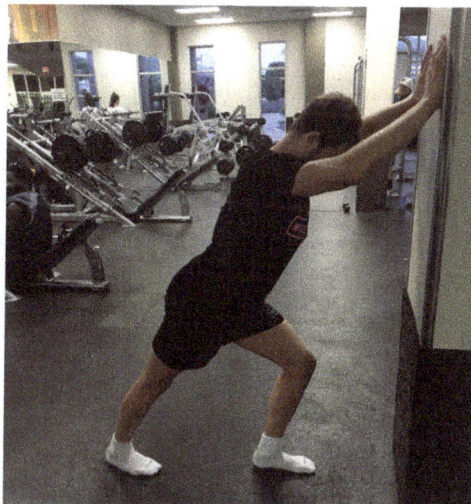

O) Arm Hang

- Grab on to a bar above your head, extend both arms, and hang.

- You should feel the stretch in your shoulders, traps, upper back, and bicep tendons.

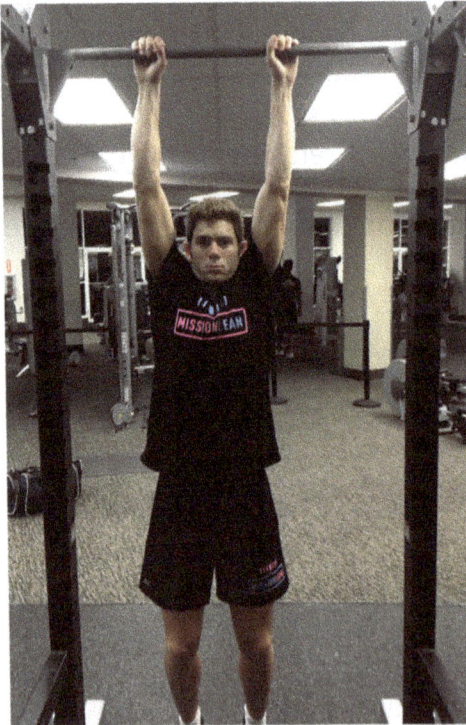

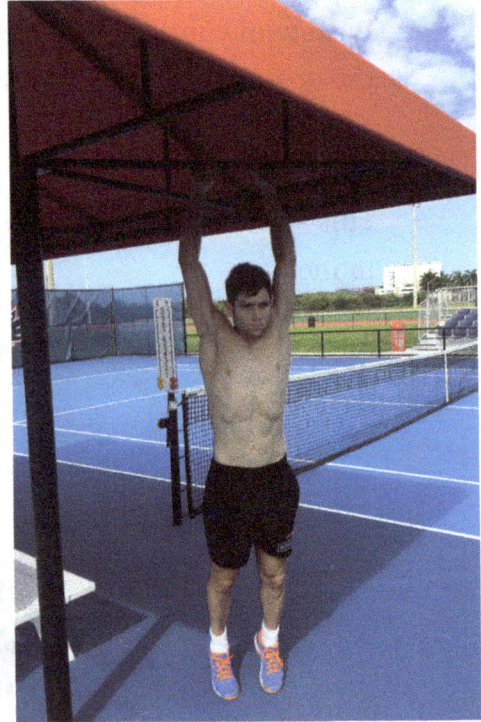

P) Bicep Tendon

- Place one arm behind you on a wall or pole, your elbow bent and your forearm resting against the surface, perpendicular to the ground. Your elbow should be positioned at roughly the same height as your shoulder.

- Rotate your feet and turn yourself towards the opposite side. Lean your body into the position so that you feel the stretch in your shoulder and bicep tendon.

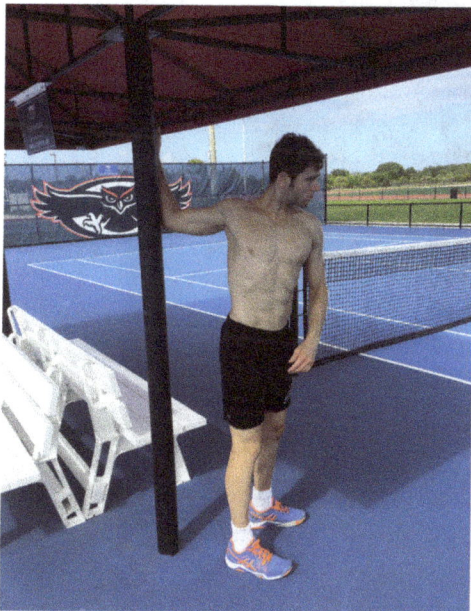

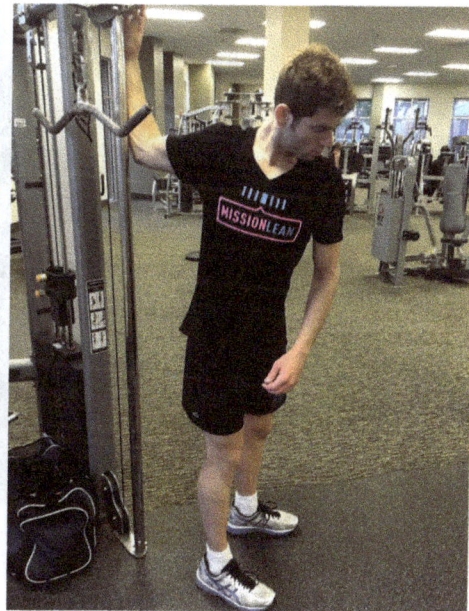

Q) Arm Across

- Standing up, bring one arm across your body and the other arm around it, so that you're hugging the crossed arm into your body.

- Pull inwards until you feel a stretch at the top of the crossed arm and shoulder.

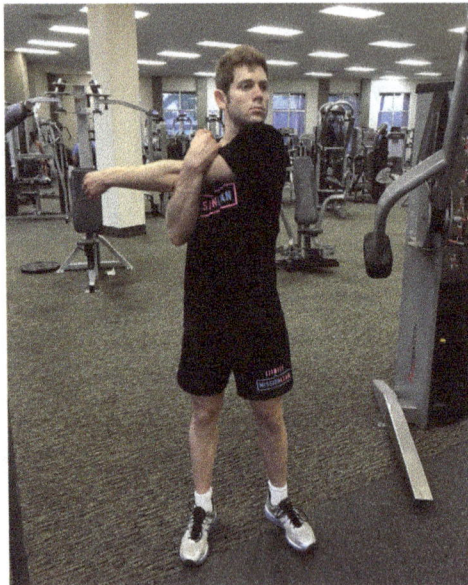

R) Arm Over Shoulder

- Bring one arm up and over the same shoulder.

- Use your opposite arm to pull the bent arm as far back as possible.

- You should feel the stretch in the triceps of the bent arm.

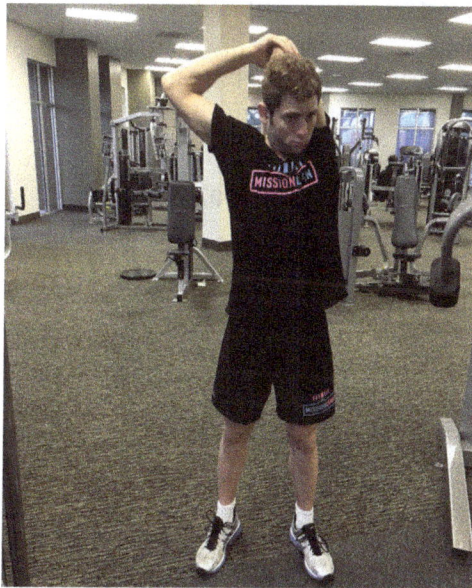

S) Roll Out with a Lacrosse Ball

- Finish off your stretching routine by rolling out your hips, butt, shoulders and upper back on a lacrosse ball.

- Lay on a matt and lean your body weight into the lacrosse ball.

- As you lean into the ball on a particular spot, move your body (slightly) up and down, and side to side, in order to massage both the targeted point and the area surrounding it.

- Use your feelings to determine when a particular area is sufficiently loose.

- Rolling out on a lacrosse ball is crucial for staying healthy because you can target small, tight areas that you can't stretch out conventionally.

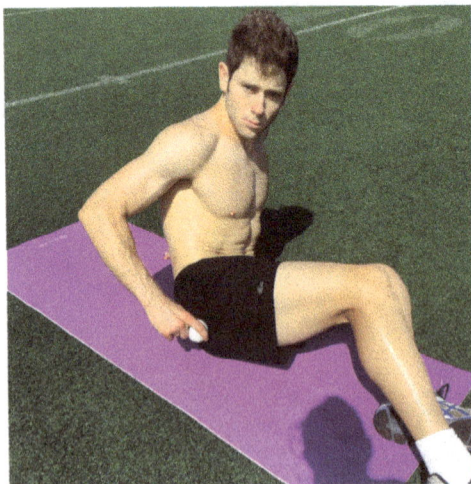

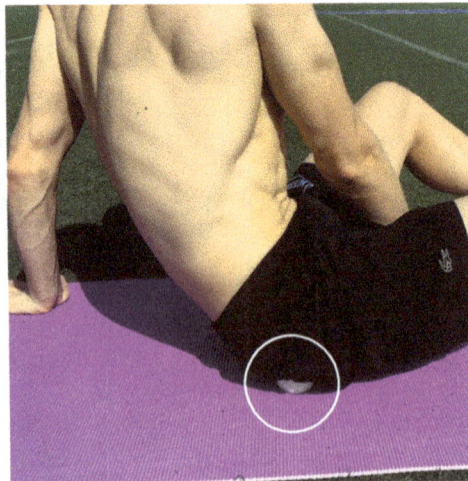

THE
4-WEEK
LEAN BODY
FITNESS
PROGRAM

The 4-Week Lean Body Fitness Program

The 4-week workout program presented here includes The Lean Body Arm and Core Workout, The Lean Body Leg and Core Workout, and running. Always be sure you follow through with The Lean Body Warm-Up before your workout and The Lean Body Stretching Routine after you've finished.

This 4-week program is complete, and gives you six workouts that should be followed Monday through Saturday. You will rest on Sunday, but if you have extra time you should stretch your body out for 15-20 minutes to assist your body in recuperating for the next week of training. If you are forced to skip a workout on a given day, simply pick up the program with the prescribed workout on the following day.

"Running" in the program means that you should run between 20 and 30 minutes at roughly a 70% pace of your maximum (feel it out during the first week or two until you hit the perfect pace, one that's manageable but where you feel youself working). Follow the tips in Chapter 2 of the book to maximize your running workout.

One point to note here is that the strength workout routines in *The Lean Body Manual* are geared towards lesser weight and more reps. Remember that the goal is to get lean, and so you're better off doing a solid number of reps (8 or 10) at a lesser weight than only 3 or 4 reps at a heavier one. Also, the objective is to limit the rest time between reps and sets so you're moving through the routine at a good pace—keeping your heart rate up throughout the workout is instrumental for building the lean body.

The specifications for each workout (number of reps, amount of weight, rest time, etc.) are separated into three levels—beginner, intermediate, and advanced. 4-weeks of workouts in each training routine are laid *out for each of the three fitness levels*. The difficulty of the workouts increases as you move forward in weeks. As a beginner, you may use the specifications for the intermediate and advanced levels to follow a 12-week Lean Body Program (although you will probably have to make some adjustments along the way as the difficulty increases steeply). As an intermediate, you may follow an 8-week Lean Body Program by picking up the advanced program on week 5 (again, you will likely need to modify a bit).

Always gauge your own feelings and adjust the program when necessary. General rule of thumb: it's better to do less than more so you avoid injury. If you're tired on a given day, you can still go in for your workout but just modify the training so that it's lighter (take off some reps/weight, or run for less time or at a slightly slower pace). Ultimately, you are the own moderator of your program. If you're consistent and focused, the results will eventually come, even if it takes slightly longer. You're better off staying healthy and working out consistently than getting injured and having to stop your training for weeks at a time.

The 4-Week Lean Body Fitness Program

Full Program

	Week 1	Week 2	Week 3	Week 4
Monday	Leg & Core	Arm & Core	Leg & Core	Arm & Core
Tuesday	Arm & Core	Leg & Core	Arm & Core	Leg & Core
Wednesday	Running	Running	Running	Running
Thursday	Leg & Core	Arm & Core	Leg & Core	Arm & Core
Friday	Arm & Core	Leg & Core	Arm & Core	Leg & Core
Saturday	Running	Running	Running	Running
Sunday	Rest	Rest	Rest	Rest

The Lean Body Arm and Core Workout

Beginner

Exercise	Week 1	Week 2	Week 3	Week 4
Pull-Ups	2	2	3	4
Push-Ups	4	5	6	8
Sit-Ups	8	10	12	15
45-Degree Back	8 *	8	10	10
# of Sets	3	3	3	3

Rest Between	2 Minutes	2 Minutes	2 Minutes	90 Seconds

		Week 1	Week 2	Week 3	Week 4
Military Press	Set 1	4, 45 ^	8, 45	8, 45	8, 45
Reverse Pull-Ups	Set 1	4	6	7	8
	Set 2	6, 45	6, 55	8, 55	8, 55
	Set 2	4	6	7	8
	Set 3	6, 55	6, 55	8, 55	10, 55
	Set 3	4	6	7	8
	Set 4	6, 55	8, 55	8, 55	10, 55
	Set 4	4	6	7	8
	Set 5	6, 55	8, 55	10, 55	10, 55
	Set 5	4	6	7	8

Rest Between		2 Min.	2 Min.	2 Min.	90 Sec.

* The beginner program doesn't have any weight added to the 45 Degree Back Extension.

^ When two numbers are given with a comma separating them, the first number represents the Reps and the second number represents how much weight to use (in pounds) Remember that the bar weighs 45 pounds by itself, so this first set of military press is simply the bar alone. For weight greater than 45 pounds, add the additional weight evenly on each side of the bar. Add clips if you want to secure that the weights don't move during the exercise.

		Week 1	Week 2	Week 3	Week 4
Deadlift	Set 1	6, 45	8, 45	8, 45	10, 45
	Set 2	6, 45	8, 45	8, 55	8, 65
	Set 3	6, 55	8, 55	8, 55	8, 65
	Set 4	6, 55	8, 55	8, 65	8, 85
	Set 5	8, 55	8, 65	8, 75	8, 85
Rest Between		2 Min.	2 Min.	2 Min.	90 Sec.

		Week 1	Week 2	Week 3	Week 4
Bench Press	Set 1	6, 45	8, 45	10, 45	10, 45
Push-Ups	Set 1	4	5	5	6
	Set 2	8, 45	8, 55	10, 55	10, 65
	Set 2	4	5	5	6
	Set 3	6, 55	6, 65	10, 65	10, 75
	Set 3	4	5	5	6
	Set 4	8, 55	8, 65	8, 75	10, 75
	Set 4	4	5	5	6
	Set 5	8, 55	8, 65	10, 75	6, 95
	Set 5	6	5	5	6
Rest Between		2 Min.	2 Min.	90 Sec.	90 Sec.

		Week 1	Week 2	Week 3	Week 4
Curl Press	Set 1	8, 10	10, 10	8, 15	10, 15
Arm Raises	Set 1	8, 3	6, 4	10, 4	8, 5
	Set 2	10, 10	8, 15	10, 15	10, 15
	Set 2	8, 3	8, 4	10, 4	8, 5
	Set 3	10, 10	8, 15	10, 15	8, 20
	Set 3	8, 3	8, 4	8, 5	10, 5
	Set 4	10, 10	8, 15	6, 20	8, 20
	Set 4	8, 3	8, 4	8, 5	10, 5
	Set 5	6, 15	10, 15	6, 20	8, 20
	Set 5	6, 4	10, 4	8, 5	10, 5
Rest Between		90 Sec.	90 Sec.	90 Sec.	90 Sec.

		Week 1	Week 2	Week 3	Week 4
Rows	Set 1	8, 20	8, 25	10, 30	8, 35
	Set 2	8, 25	10, 30	10, 30	10, 35
	Set 3	8, 25	10, 30	10, 35	8, 40
	Set 4	8, 30	8, 35	10, 35	10, 40
	Set 5	8, 30	8, 35	8, 40	8, 45
Rest Between		2 Min.	2 Min.	90 Sec.	90 Sec.

		Week 1	Week 2	Week 3	Week 4
Wrist Raise	Set 1	6, 2	6, 3	6, 4	6, 5
Wrist Curl	Set 1	6, 2	6, 3	6, 4	6, 5
	Set 2	8, 2	8, 3	8, 4	8, 5
	Set 2	8, 2	8, 3	8, 4	8, 5
	Set 3	8, 2	6, 4	6, 5	8, 5
	Set 3	8, 2	6, 4	6, 5	8, 5
	Set 4	6, 3	6, 4	6, 5	6, 6
	Set 4	6, 3	6, 4	6, 5	6, 6
	Set 5	8, 3	8, 4	8, 5	8, 6
	Set 5	8, 3	8, 4	8, 5	8, 6
Rest Between		90 Sec.	90 Sec.	90 Sec.	90 Sec.

Intermediate

Exercise	Week 1	Week 2	Week 3	Week 4
Pull-Ups	5	6	7	8
Push-Ups	8	10	12	12
Sit-Ups	15	18	20	25
45-Degree Back	8, 5 *	8, 5	10, 5	8, 10
# of Sets	3	3	3	3
Rest Between	90 Sec.	90 Sec.	90 Sec.	90 Sec.

		Week 1	Week 2	Week 3	Week 4
Military Press	Set 1	8, 45 ^	10, 45	10, 45	10, 45
Reverse Pull-Ups	Set 1	8	9	10	10
	Set 2	8, 55	10, 55	10, 65	10, 65
	Set 2	8	9	10	10
	Set 3	8, 55	8, 65	10, 65	10, 65
	Set 3	8	9	10	10
	Set 4	10, 55	8, 65	8, 75	8, 75
	Set 4	8	9	10	10
	Set 5	10, 55	8, 65	8, 75	10, 75
	Set 5	8	9	10	10
Rest Between		90 Sec.	90 Sec.	90 Sec.	90 Sec.

*When two numbers are given with a comma separating them, the first number represents the Reps and the second number represents how much weight to use (in pounds). For the 45 Degree Back Extension exercise, use a weight plate and hold it to your chest with both arms crossed over.

^ Remember that the bar weighs 45 pounds by itself, so this first set of military press is using the bar alone. For weight greater than 45 pounds, add the additional weight evenly on each side of the bar. Add clips if you want to secure that the weights don't move during the exercise.

Deadlift		Week 1	Week 2	Week 3	Week 4
	Set 1	10, 45	10, 45	8, 65	8, 95
	Set 2	8, 65	8, 65	8, 85	8, 95
	Set 3	8, 65	8, 85	8, 95	8, 105
	Set 4	8, 85	8, 85	8, 95	8, 105
	Set 5	8, 85	8, 95	8, 105	8, 115
Rest Between		90 Sec.	90 Sec.	90 Sec.	90 Sec.

Bench Press / Push-Ups		Week 1	Week 2	Week 3	Week 4
Bench Press	Set 1	10, 45	10, 45	12, 45	12, 45
Push-Ups	Set 1	6	6	8	8
	Set 2	10, 65	10, 85	10, 95	10, 95
	Set 2	6	8	8	8
	Set 3	10, 85	8, 95	10, 95	10, 95
	Set 3	8	8	8	10
	Set 4	8, 95	10, 95	8, 115	10, 115
	Set 4	8	8	10	10
	Set 5	8, 95	10, 95	8, 115	10, 115
	Set 5	8	8	10	10
Rest Between		90 Sec.	90 Sec.	90 Sec.	90 Sec.

Curl Press / Arm Raises		Week 1	Week 2	Week 3	Week 4
Curl Press	Set 1	8, 15	8, 20	10, 20	8, 25
Arm Raises	Set 1	8, 5	10, 5	8, 6	8, 8
	Set 2	10, 15	10, 20	8, 25	10, 25
	Set 2	8, 5	10, 5	10, 6	8, 8
	Set 3	8, 20	8, 25	10, 25	10, 25
	Set 3	10, 5	8, 6	10, 6	8, 8
	Set 4	8, 20	8, 25	10, 25	6, 30
	Set 4	10, 5	8, 6	10, 6	8, 8
	Set 5	10, 20	8, 25	10, 25	6, 30
	Set 5	10, 5	8, 6	10, 6	10, 8
Rest Between		90 Sec.	90 Sec.	90 Sec.	90 Sec.

		Week 1	Week 2	Week 3	Week 4
Rows	Set 1	8, 35	10, 40	10, 45	8, 50
	Set 2	10, 35	10, 40	8, 50	8, 55
	Set 3	8, 40	8, 45	10, 50	10, 55
	Set 4	10, 40	10, 45	8, 55	10, 60
	Set 5	8, 45	8, 50	10, 55	10, 65
Rest Between		90 Sec.	90 Sec.	90 Sec.	90 Sec.

		Week 1	Week 2	Week 3	Week 4
Wrist Raise	Set 1	6, 5	8, 6	10, 6	8, 8
Wrist Curl	Set 1	6, 5	8, 6	10, 6	8, 8
	Set 2	8, 5	8, 6	6, 8	8, 8
	Set 2	8, 5	8, 6	6, 8	8, 8
	Set 3	8, 5	10, 6	6, 8	8, 8
	Set 3	8, 5	10, 6	6, 8	8, 8
	Set 4	6, 6	10, 6	6, 8	10, 8
	Set 4	6, 6	10, 6	6, 8	10, 8
	Set 5	8, 6	10, 6	8, 8	10, 8
	Set 5	8, 6	10, 6	8, 8	10, 8
Rest Between		90 Sec.	90 Sec.	90 Sec.	90 Sec.

Advanced

Exercise	Week 1	Week 2	Week 3	Week 4
Pull-Ups	10	10	12	12
Push-Ups	12	15	15	16
Sit-Ups	25	30	35	40
45-Degree Back	10, 10*	10, 10	12, 10	12, 10
# of Sets	3	3	3	3
Rest Between	90 Sec.	90 Sec.	90 Sec.	90 Sec.

		Week 1	Week 2	Week 3	Week 4
Military Press	Set 1	10, 45 ^	10, 45	12, 45	12, 45
Reverse Pull-Ups	Set 1	10	12	15	15
	Set 2	10, 65	10, 65	12, 65	12, 65
	Set 2	10	12	15	15
	Set 3	10, 65	10, 75	10, 85	10, 85
	Set 3	10	12	15	15
	Set 4	8, 75	8, 85	10, 85	10, 85
	Set 4	10	12	15	15
	Set 5	10, 75	8, 85	10, 85	6, 95
	Set 5	10	12	15	15
Rest Between		90 Sec.	90 Sec.	90 Sec.	90 Sec.

* When two numbers are given with a comma separating them, the first number represents the Reps and the second number represents how much weight to use (in pounds). For the 45 Degree Back Extension exercise, use a weight plate and hold it to your chest with both arms crossed over.

^ Remember that the bar weighs 45 pounds by itself, so this first set of military press is simply the bar alone. For weight greater than 45 pounds, add the additional weight evenly on each side of the bar. Add clips if you want to secure that the weights don't move during the exercise.

Deadlift		Week 1	Week 2	Week 3	Week 4
	Set 1	8, 95	8, 95	10, 95	10, 95
	Set 2	8, 95	8, 115	8, 135	8, 135
	Set 3	8, 105	8, 135	8, 135	8, 135
	Set 4	8, 105	8, 135	8, 135	8, 155
	Set 5	8, 115	8, 135	8, 135	8, 155
Rest Between		90 Sec.	90 Sec.	90 Sec.	90 Sec.

Bench Press Push-Ups		Week 1	Week 2	Week 3	Week 4
	Set 1	12, 45	12, 45	10, 90	10, 90
	Set 1	8	10	10	10
	Set 2	8, 95	10, 95	10, 135	10, 135
	Set 2	8	10	10	10
	Set 3	10, 95	8, 135	10, 135	10, 145
	Set 3	8	10	10	12
	Set 4	6, 135	8, 135	10, 135	10, 155
	Set 4	10	10	10	12
	Set 5	6, 135	10, 135	8, 145	6, 175
	Set 5	10	10	10	12
Rest Between		90 Sec.	90 Sec.	90 Sec.	90 Sec.

Curl Press Arm Raises		Week 1	Week 2	Week 3	Week 4
	Set 1	8, 25	10, 25	8, 30	8, 30
	Set 1	8, 8	10, 8	10, 10	10, 10
	Set 2	10, 25	8, 30	10, 30	10, 30
	Set 2	8, 8	10, 8	10, 10	10, 10
	Set 3	10, 25	8, 30	10, 30	8, 35
	Set 3	8, 8	8, 10	10, 10	10, 10
	Set 4	10, 25	8, 30	10, 30	8, 35
	Set 4	8, 8	8, 10	10, 10	10, 10
	Set 5	6, 30	8, 30	6, 35	10, 35
	Set 5	10, 8	10, 10	10, 10	10, 10
Rest Between		90 Sec.	90 Sec.	90 Sec.	90 Sec.

Rows		Week 1	Week 2	Week 3	Week 4
	Set 1	8, 50	10, 60	10, 70	10, 75
	Set 2	8, 55	10, 60	10, 75	8, 85
	Set 3	10, 55	8, 70	10, 75	10, 85
	Set 4	10, 60	10, 70	8, 85	8, 90
	Set 5	10, 65	8, 75	8, 85	8, 100
Rest Between		90 Sec.	90 Sec.	90 Sec.	90 Sec.

		Week 1	Week 2	Week 3	Week 4
Wrist Raise	Set 1	8, 8	8, 10	10, 10	8, 12
Wrist Curl	Set 1	8, 8	8, 10	10, 10	8, 12
	Set 2	10, 8	8, 10	8, 12	10, 12
	Set 2	10, 8	8, 10	8, 12	10, 12
	Set 3	10, 8	10, 10	8, 12	10, 12
	Set 3	10, 8	10, 10	8, 12	10, 12
	Set 4	10, 8	10, 10	8, 12	10, 12
	Set 4	10, 8	10, 10	8, 12	10, 12
	Set 5	8, 10	8, 12	10, 12	10, 12
	Set 5	8, 10	8, 12	10, 12	10, 12
Rest Between		90 Sec.	90 Sec.	90 Sec.	90 Sec.

The Lean Body Leg and Core Workout

Beginner

Exercise		Week 1	Week 2	Week 3	Week 4
Squats	Set 1	2, 45 *	4, 45	6, 45	8, 45
Squat Jumps	Set 1	2	4	4	6
	Set 2	2, 45	4, 55	6, 65	6, 85
	Set 2	2	4	4	6
	Set 3	2, 55	4, 65	4, 75	8, 85
	Set 3	2	4	4	8
	Set 4	2, 55	4,65	6,75	8, 85
	Set 4	3	4	6	8
	Set 5	2, 55	4,65	6, 75	8, 95
	Set 5	4	4	6	8
Rest Between		2 Min.	2 Min.	2 Min.	2 Min.

* When two numbers are given with a comma separating them, the first number represents the Reps and the second number represents how much weight to use (in pounds). Remember that the bar weighs 45 pounds by itself, so this first set of squats is simply the bar alone. For weight greater than 45 pounds, add the additional weight evenly on each side of the bar. Add clips if you want to secure that the weights don't move during the exercise.

Lunges	Set 1	2, 45 ^	4, 45	6, 45	8, 45
Lunge Jumps	Set 1	4	6	8	10
	Set 2	2, 45	4, 55	8, 55	6, 75
	Set 2	4	6	8	10
	Set 3	2, 45	4, 55	6, 65	8, 75
	Set 3	6	8	8	10
	Set 4	2, 45	6, 55	6, 65	8, 75
	Set 4	6	8	10	12
	Set 5	2, 45	6, 55	8, 65	10, 75
	Set 5	8	8	10	12
Rest Between		2 Min.	2 Min.	2 Min.	2 Min.

^ Each Rep is one lunge with a single leg. Reps will always be given in even numbers, so complete the same number on each leg. Complete all of your Reps on one leg before moving to the other.

Plank	Set 1	15 Sec.	20 Sec.	25 Sec.	30 Sec.
Superman	Set 1	15 Sec.	20 Sec.	25 Sec.	30 Sec.
Bicycles	Set 1	10	15	20	25
	Set 2	15 Sec.	20 Sec.	25 Sec.	30 Sec.
	Set 2	15 Sec.	20 Sec.	25 Sec.	30 Sec.
	Set 2	10	15	20	25
	Set 3	15 Sec.	20 Sec.	25 Sec.	30 Sec.
	Set 3	15 Sec.	20 Sec.	25 Sec.	30 Sec.
	Set 3	10	15	20	25
Rest Between		2 Min.	90 Sec.	90 Sec.	90 Sec.

Leg Raises	Set 1	4, 15	4, 20	6, 25	8, 30
	Set 2	4, 15	4, 20	8, 25	6, 35
	Set 3	4, 20	6, 25	6, 30	8, 35
	Set 4	4, 20	6, 25	8, 30	8, 40
Rest Between		90 Sec.	90 Sec.	90 Sec.	90 Sec.

Swiss Ball	Set 1	4	6	8	10
	Set 2	4	6	8	10
	Set 3	6	8	10	12
	Set 4	6	8	10	12
Rest Between		90 Sec.	60 Sec.	60 Sec.	60 Sec.

Calf Raises	Set 1	6, 20	6, 30	8, 35	8, 45
	Set 2	6, 20	6, 30	8, 40	8, 50
	Set 3	6, 20	6, 35	8, 40	8, 50
	Set 4	8, 20	8, 35	8, 45	8, 55
Rest Between		90 Sec.	90 Sec.	90 Sec.	90 Sec.

Intermediate

Exercise		Week 1	Week 2	Week 3	Week 4
Squats	Set 1	10, 45 *	12, 45	12, 45	12, 45
Squat Jumps	Set 1	6	8	10	12
	Set 2	8, 95	8, 105	8, 95	10, 95
	Set 2	6	8	10	12
	Set 3	8, 95	8, 115	8, 135	8, 135
	Set 3	8	8	10	12
	Set 4	8, 105	8, 115	8, 135	8, 155
	Set 4	8	10	10	12
	Set 5	8, 105	8, 135 ^	8, 155	8, 165
	Set 5	8	10	10	12
Rest Between		2 Min.	90 Sec.	90 Sec.	90 Sec.

* When two numbers are given with a comma separating them, the first number represents the Reps and the second number represents how much weight to use (in pounds). Remember that the bar weighs 45 pounds by itself, so this first set of squats is simply the bar alone. For weight greater than 45 pounds, add the additional weight evenly on each side of the bar. Add clips if you want to secure that the weights don't move during the exercise.

^ This is the first set of Reps where you will have two 45 pound plates on either side.

Lunges	Set 1	10, 45 †	10, 45	12, 45	16, 45
Lunge Jumps	Set 1	10	12	16	18
	Set 2	6, 65	10, 65	12, 65	16, 65
	Set 2	10	16	16	18
	Set 3	6, 75	10, 75	12, 75	12, 95
	Set 3	10	16	16	20
	Set 4	8, 75	12, 75	12, 85	12, 95
	Set 4	12	16	18	20
	Set 5	10, 75	12, 75	12, 85	16, 95
	Set 5	12	16	18	20
Rest Between		2 Min.	2 Min.	90 Sec.	90 Sec.

† Each Rep is one lunge with a single leg. Reps will always be given in even numbers, so complete the same number on each leg. Complete all of your Reps on one leg before moving to the other.

Plank	Set 1	30 Sec.	30 Sec.	45 Sec.	45 Sec.
Superman	Set 1	30 Sec.	30 Sec.	45 Sec.	45 Sec.
Bicycles	Set 1	25	35	45	50
	Set 2	30 Sec.	30 Sec.	45 Sec.	45 Sec.
	Set 2	30 Sec.	30 Sec.	45 Sec.	45 Sec.
	Set 2	25	35	50	50
	Set 3	30 Sec.	30 Sec.	45 Sec.	45 Sec.
	Set 3	30 Sec.	30 Sec.	45 Sec.	45 Sec.
	Set 3	25	45	50	50
Rest Between		90 Sec.	90 Sec.	60 Sec.	60 Sec.

Leg Raises	Set 1	8, 30	8, 40	8, 45	8, 55
	Set 2	8, 35	10, 45	8, 55	10, 55
	Set 3	8, 40	8, 50	10, 55	10, 60
	Set 4	10, 40	10, 50	8, 60	10, 65
Rest Between		90 Sec.	90 Sec.	90 Sec.	90 Sec.

Swiss Ball	Set 1	10	12	12	15
	Set 2	10	12	15	15
	Set 3	12	15	15	18
	Set 4	12	15	18	18
Rest Between		60 Sec.	60 Sec.	60 Sec.	60 Sec.

Calf Raises	Set 1	8, 45	8, 50	10, 50	10, 60
	Set 2	8, 50	8, 60	10, 60	10, 70
	Set 3	8, 55	8, 65	10, 65	10, 70
	Set 4	8, 60	8, 70	10, 70	10, 80
Rest Between		90 Sec.	90 Sec.	90 Sec.	90 Sec.

Advanced

Exercise		Week 1	Week 2	Week 3	Week 4
Squats	Set 1	12, 45 *	12, 45	12, 95	12, 95
Squat Jumps	Set 1	10	12	12	12
	Set 2	10, 95	10, 135	12, 135	12, 135
	Set 2	10	12	12	12
	Set 3	8, 135 ^	10, 135	12, 135	12, 155
	Set 3	10	12	12	12
	Set 4	8, 155	10, 155	12, 155	10, 185
	Set 4	10	12	12	12
	Set 5	8, 165	10, 185	10, 185	10, 225
	Set 5	10	12	12	12
Rest Between		2 Min.	2 Min.	2 Min.	90 Sec.

* When two numbers are given with a comma separating them, the first number represents the Reps and the second number represents how much weight to use (in pounds). Remember that the bar weighs 45 pounds by itself, so this first set of squats is simply the bar alone. For weight greater than 45 pounds, add the additional weight evenly on each side of the bar. Add clips if you want to secure that the weights don't move during the exercise.

^ This is the first set of Reps where you will have two 45 pound plates on either side.

Lunges	Set 1	16, 45 †	16, 45	20, 45	20, 45
Lunge Jumps	Set 1	18	20	30	40
	Set 2	16, 65	16, 65	16, 85	16, 95
	Set 2	18	24	30	40
	Set 3	12, 95	16, 95	16, 95	16, 95
	Set 3	20	26	35	40
	Set 4	12, 95	16, 95	16, 105	16, 115
	Set 4	20	28	35	40
	Set 5	14, 95	16, 95	16, 105	16, 115
	Set 5	20	30	40	40
Rest Between		2 Min.	2 Min.	90 Sec.	90 Sec.

† Each Rep is one lunge with a single leg. Reps will always be given in even numbers, so complete the same number on each leg. Complete all of your Reps on one leg before moving to the other.

Plank	Set 1	45 Sec.	45 Sec.	1 Min.	1 Min.
Superman	Set 1	45 Sec.	45 Sec.	1 Min.	1 Min.
Bicycles	Set 1	50	50	55	60
	Set 2	45 Sec.	45 Sec.	1 Min.	1 Min.
	Set 2	45 Sec.	45 Sec.	1 Min.	1 Min.
	Set 2	50	50	60	65
	Set 3	45 Sec.	45 Sec.	1 Min.	1 Min.
	Set 3	45 Sec.	45 Sec.	1 Min.	1 Min.
	Set 3	50	50	60	70
Rest Between		60 Sec.	60 Sec.	45 Sec.	30 Sec.

Leg Raises	Set 1	8, 50	10, 60	10, 70	10, 70
	Set 2	10, 55	10, 70	10, 85	10, 90
	Set 3	10, 65	10, 75	10, 90	10, 90
	Set 4	10, 70	10, 80	10, 90	10, 100
Rest Between		90 Sec.	90 Sec.	90 Sec.	90 Sec.

Swiss Ball	Set 1	12	12	18	18
	Set 2	15	18	18	18
	Set 3	18	18	20	22
	Set 4	18	20	20	25
Rest Between		60 Sec.	60 Sec.	60 Sec.	60 Sec.

Calf Raises	Set 1	10, 60	10, 70	10, 85	10, 90
	Set 2	10, 70	10,85	10, 90	10, 90
	Set 3	10, 75	10, 85	10, 100	10, 110
	Set 4	10, 80	10, 90	10, 100	10, 120
Rest Between		90 Sec.	90 Sec.	90 Sec.	90 Sec.

PART V:
THE LEAN BODY
MEAL PLAN

THE LEAN BODY DIET
MODUS OPERANDI

The Lean Body Diet: Modus Operandi

Diet and health cookbooks make it seem like eating healthy and preparing your own food is extremely complicated and involved. It's not. Doing it right is simple: you should be consuming natural, single-ingredient, and (ideally) organic foods. Once you start following a logical and sustainable nutritional approach, the lean body will be well within reach.

What *not* to eat.

- Dairy: Yogurt, Milk, Cheese
- Wheat: Bread, Wheat Pasta
- Soy
- "Gluten-free" Products
  (you will buy pure grains that
  do not contain gluten)
- Canned Foods
- Deli Meats
  (which are heavily processed)
- Eggs

What you do eat.

Grains and Beans

- Brown Rice
- Wild (Black) Rice
- Buckwheat
- Rice Pasta
- Quinoa
- Steel Cut Oats
- Yellow/Green Lentils
- Kidney beans

Vegetables

- Broccoli
- Cauliflower
- Cabbage (Red & Green)
- Bok choy
- Chard (Red & Green)
- Onion/Garlic/Scallion/Shallot
- Zucchini
- Squash
- Spinach
- Lettuce
- Avocado
- Carrots
- Celery
- Cucumber
- Kale
- Dandelion Greens
- Ginger root
- Beets
- Peppers
- Tomatoes
- Eggplant
- Mushrooms

Chicken & Fish

- Wild Fish — Salmon, Yellowtail, Snapper, Sea Bass, Tuna, Sardines (try to buy low mercury fish)
- Chicken Breast
- Lean Red Meat (avoid ground beef)

Fruits

- Grapefruit
- Orange

- Grapes
- Apples
- Pears
- Bananas
- Strawberries
- Blueberries
- Raspberries
- Blackberries
- Peaches
- Nectarines
- Plums

Spices (be sure not to over-salt your food)

- Black Pepper
- Sea Salt
- Cumin
- Oregano
- Turmeric
- Cardamom
- Coriander
- Cayenne Pepper
- Cinnamon
- Mustard Seed
- Red Pepper Flakes

Nuts, Dried Fruit, and Dark Chocolate

- Brazil nuts
- Walnuts
- Almonds
- Hazelnuts
- Pistachios (unsalted)
- Pecans
- Raisins
- Figs
- Dates
- 85% Dark Chocolate

Oils and Vinegar

- Olive Oil
- Balsamic Vinegar
- Apple Cider Vinegar

Equipment

- Large Stir-fry Pan with Lid
- Large Boiling Pot
- Steaming Basket for Pot
- Mid-Size Pot for Boiling Grains
- Vitamix Blender
- Toaster

Execution

Breakfast:

- Oatmeal eaten alongside nuts, dark chocolate, dried fruit, and fresh fruit.

- Slice of Mestemacher or Dimpflmeier bread with sliced fresh fruit on top.

- Vitamix Smoothies (later explained)

Lunch and Dinner:

- Should be comprised of 50% grains, 30% vegetables and healthy fat (avocado), and 20% protein (fish, chicken, or lean red meat). Try to eat chicken and red meat each once per week, and low mercury fish twice per week.

- Vegetables should either be steamed, grilled, or sautéed in light olive oil. You can also eat them raw.

- Grains and rice pasta should be boiled.

- Fish can be cooked in the oven, steamed, or grilled. Chicken and lean red meat can be prepared in the oven, on the grill, or in a "stir-fry" with olive oil and vegetables.

- Vary the grains and vegetables you eat every day.

- Salads are a great option in place of cooked vegetables. Quinoa is a perfect grain to toss directly into the salad.

- Soups can be made with beans, quinoa, and vegetables.

Dessert:

- Frozen banana. Allow bananas to ripen until brown, peel, and store in the freezer. Add fresh fruit, dried fruit, berries, nuts, and 85% dark chocolate.

- Dates, figs, nuts, and dark chocolate, alongside fresh fruit. Find your perfect combination.

- Tip: to jump-start your lean body program, always include banana in your dessert. This will fill you up so you don't overeat nuts and dried fruit, which are highly caloric.

Snacks:

- Fresh fruit (apple, banana, orange, pear)
- Celery
- Carrots
- Vitamix Smoothie

Vitamix Smoothie:

- Base of Vitamix is water and *frozen* banana

- Add raw vegetables and fruit: carrots, celery, kale, broccoli, apple, pear, etc.

- Experiment and find your go-to recipe.

Preparation:

- When you prepare batches of grains, make extra and store leftovers in the refrigerator (grains take the most time to cook out of all the food listed). Having pre-cooked grains accessible will allow for easy and quick preparation of your meals.

- Make sure to always have fruits and vegetables in your home. Designate specific days of the week to go shopping so that you never come home to an empty kitchen.

LEAN BODY
RECIPES

Lean Body Recipes

The following is a list of delicious, lean body recipes for breakfast, lunch, dinner, and snacks. Refer to The 4-Week Lean Body Meal Plan for a detailed plan of action for what to eat when. The recipes below don't include red meat and chicken, but do include fish. Replacing meat with fish (and including vegetarian meals) at the beginning of your program will get you results quicker. After a month or two, once your lean body efforts have started to take form, you can begin incorporating chicken and red meat back into your program, each once per week (and reduce your fish intake to twice per week).

LEAN BODY BREAKFAST RECIPES

1. FRUIT "JAM" ON TOAST

10 Minutes

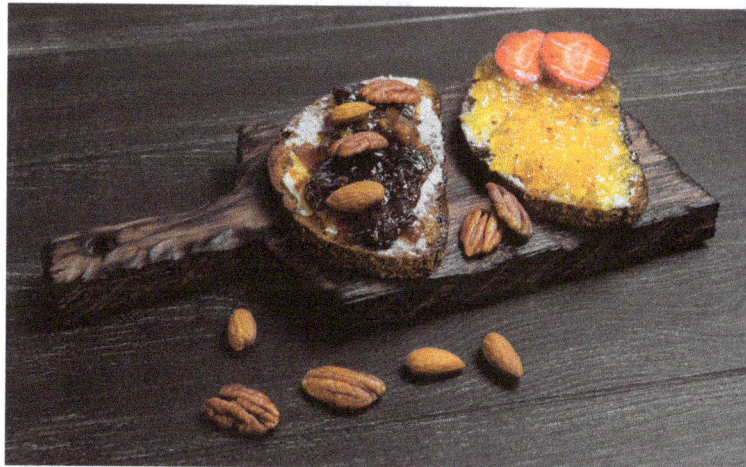

Ingredients:

1 Slice Mestemacher
or Dimpflmeier Bread

3 Large Dried Medjool Dates

3-4 Dried Apricots

1/8 cup Raisins

1/8 cup Almonds

1-2 Fresh Strawberries

Directions:

1. Toast a slice of bread.

2. Slice dried dates and apricots in half. Wash and slice strawberries too.

3. Place the dried fruit on the bread and apply pressure. The heat of the warm toast will allow you to spread the fruit like a jam.

4. Place dates on ½ of the slice and apricots on the other ½.

5. Sprinkle on raisins and almonds.

6. Add fresh strawberries for extra flavor.

2. OATMEAL WITH WALNUTS, BERRIES & CINNAMON

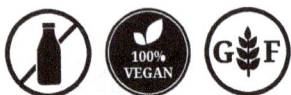

⏱ 15 Minutes

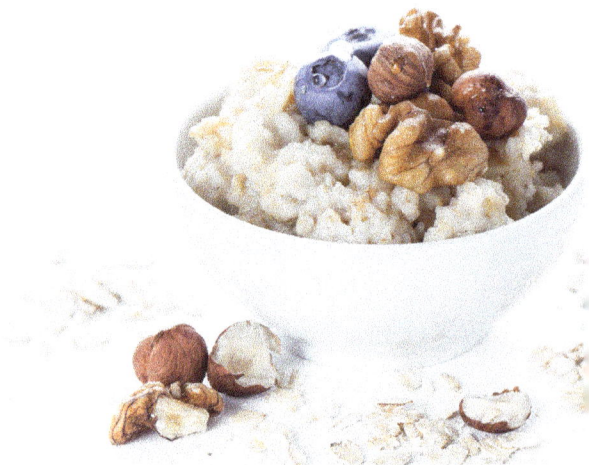

Ingredients:

¼ cup Steel Cut Oats

¼ cup Blueberries

5-6 Walnuts & Hazelnuts

Directions:

1. Bring ¾ cup of water to a boil.

2. Pour in oats and cook for 12-15 minutes (or until you achieve your preferred texture.)

3. Allow to cool for 5 minutes.

4. Place in a bowl, add blueberries, walnuts and hazelnuts. Optional: You can chop up the nuts before mixing them in.

3. OATMEAL & FRESH FRUIT

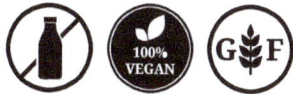

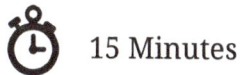 15 Minutes

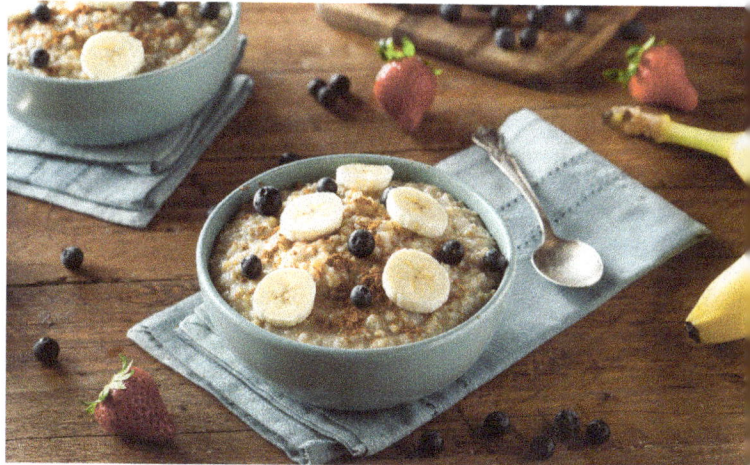

Ingredients:

¼ Cup Organic Steel Cut Oats

½ Banana

¼ Cup Blueberries

Cinnamon

Directions:

1. Boil ¾ cup water for the oats.

2. Cook oats for 12-15 minutes.

3. Mix and allow to cool for a few minutes.

4. Slice up banana.

5. Serve in a bowl and add banana, blueberries and cinnamon to taste.

4. BREAKFAST TOAST

10 Minutes

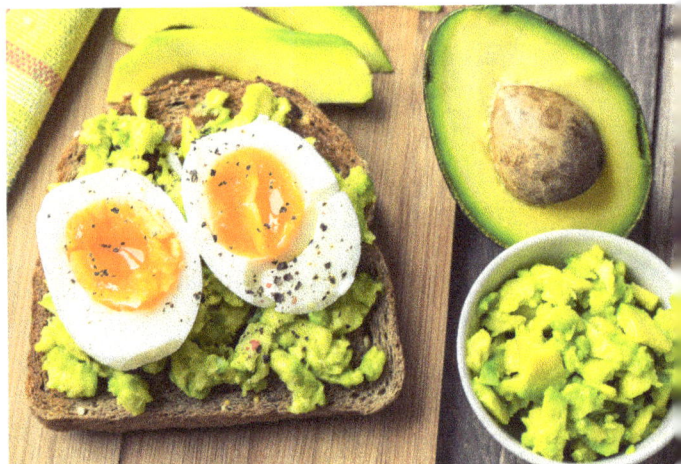

Ingredients:

1 Egg (Optional: If you're used to eating eggs, you can include—otherwise just use avocado on the toast. Ultimately, you want to rid eggs from your diet but I have included the egg here as a transitional recipe.)

1 Slice of Mestemacher or Dimpflmeier

¼ Avocado

Salt & Pepper

Directions:

1. Boil the egg for 10 minutes.

2. Toast slice of Mestemacher.

3. Use avocado as a "butter" and apply liberally to the slice.

4. Remove the egg's shell, slice up the egg into as many or as few pieces as you like and place on top of the toast.

5. Salt and pepper to taste.

5. BEET SMOOTHIE

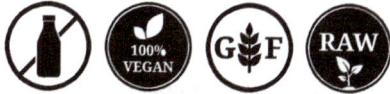

⊘ 🌱 100% VEGAN G F RAW

⏱ 5 Minutes

Ingredients:

1 Beet
Fresh Ginger
½ Apple
4-5 Brocolli Florets
2 Leaves of Chard

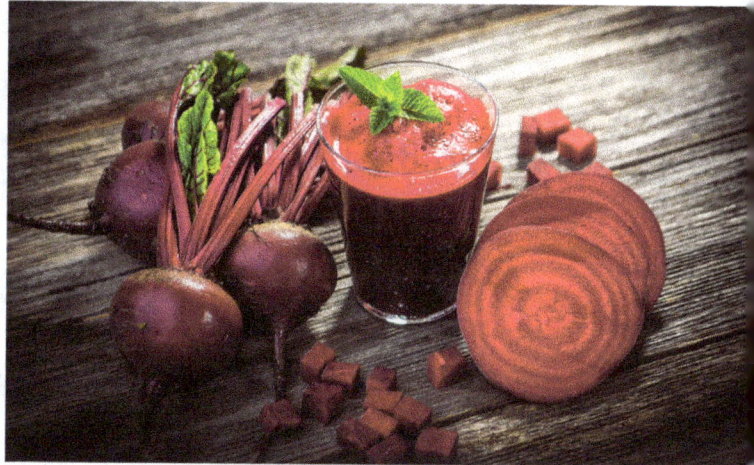

Directions:

1. Wash and peel uncooked beet and ginger.

2. Wash apple, broccoli, and chard.

3. Chop up all vegetables and place into blender (Vitamix is ideal).

4. Add water and ice, and blend. Drink immediately.

6. BUCKWHEAT PANCAKES

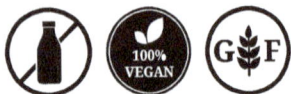

10 Minutes

Ingredients:

1/2 Cup Buckwheat Flour

1/2 Very Ripe and Sweet
Banana—Mashed

½ Cup Apple Sauce

Pinch of Baking Soda

Olive Oil

½ Cup Water

Organic Maple Syrup

Fresh Berries

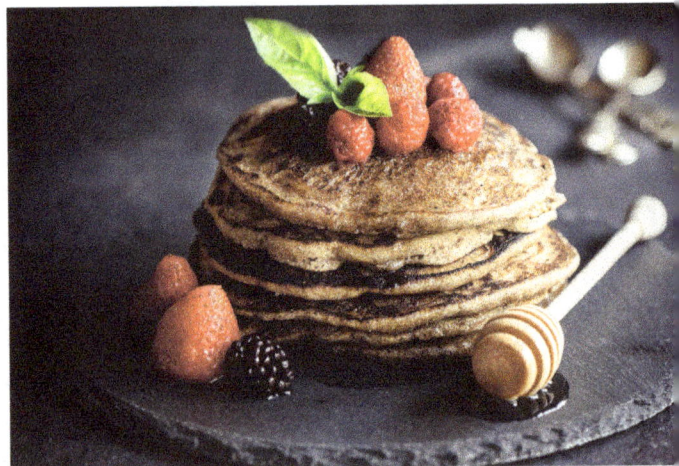

Directions:

1. Mix flour, apple sauce, water, mashed banana and baking soda in a bowl.

2. Whip contents of the bowl until they are a dense but malleable consistency. You should be able to pour the batter, but it should still be dense (almost like putty).

3. Heat up olive oil on a skillet and wait until it is very hot. Test this by throwing some water—if it evaporates immediately, then it is sufficiently hot.

4. Pour mixture into skillet in 5" batches.

5. Cook on each side for 1 minute.

6. Add fresh berries and 2 Tbsp. of maple syrup.

LEAN BODY LUNCH RECIPES

1. FRESH VEGETABLE SALAD

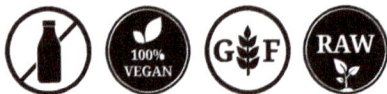

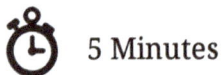 5 Minutes

Ingredients:

2 Slices Romaine

2 Radishes

4-5 Cherry Tomatoes

¼ Red Pepper

¼ Yellow Pepper

¼ Yellow Onion

½ Whole Avocado

1 tbsp. Olive Oil

2 tbsp. Balsamic Vinegar

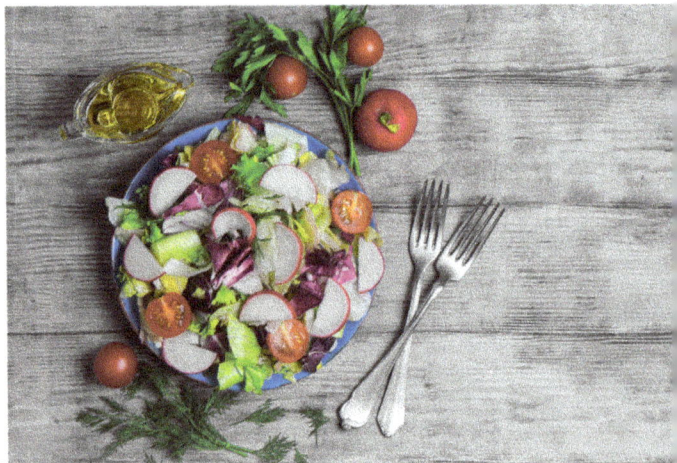

Directions:

1. Wash and thinly slice all vegetables. Place in bowl.

2. Wash avocado. Cut in half, remove seed and skin, and slice thinly. Add to salad.

3. Add olive oil and vinegar.

4. Add protein if you want: grilled fish, canned tuna or sardines (add lemon for taste), or chicken breast.

5. Mix and enjoy.

2. BAKED COD & VEGGIES

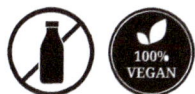

20 Minutes

Ingredients:

1/2 Medium Sweet Potato
1/2 Medium Potato
1 Large Carrot
¼ Squash
2-3 Broccoli Florets
1/3 lb. Cod
Olive Oil
Cayenne
Salt
Lemon (for taste)

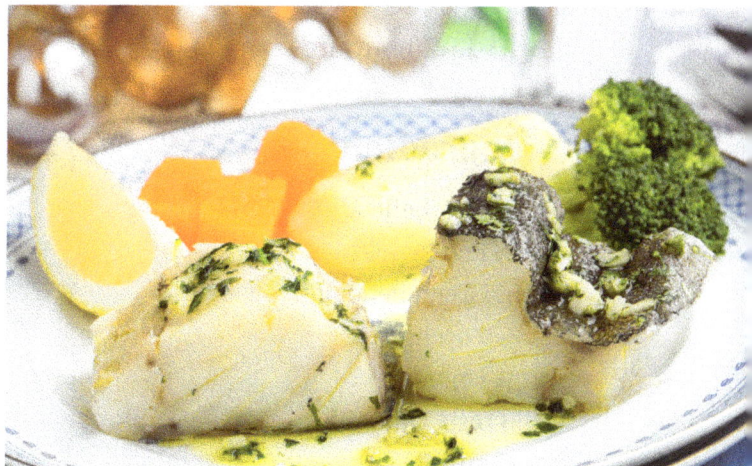

Directions:

1. Preheat oven to 400 degrees.

2. Wash and cut potatoes into quarters.

3. Wash carrot and broccoli. Cut into thin pieces.

4. Cover baking dish in olive oil. Use brush to be consistent.

5. Place vegetables into baking dish.

6. Place cod into baking dish.

7. Drizzle with olive oil.

8. Add Cayenne and salt to taste.

9. Bake for 15-20 minutes.

3. STUFFED MUSHROOMS

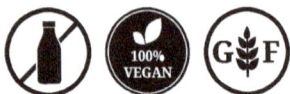

⏱ 20 Minutes

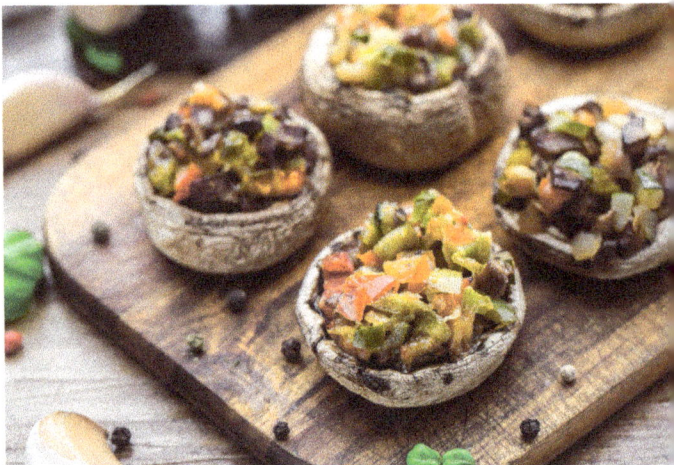

Ingredients:

2 Portobello Mushroom Caps

½ Red Pepper

½ Green Pepper

¼ Zucchini

½ Onion

3 tbsp. Olive Oil

Cumin

Salt & Pepper

Directions:

1. Wash mushroom caps and remove the stems.

2. Wash and finely chop the mushroom stems, peppers, zucchini, and onions.

3. Sautee the veggies in a pan with 1 tbsp. olive oil for about 10 minutes.

4. Add salt, pepper and cumin for flavor.

5. Preheat oven to 350 degrees.

6. Drizzle 1 tbsp. olive oil over baking dish.

7. Use brush to cover mushroom caps with olive oil.

8. Use tablespoon to generously stuff the caps with sautéed vegetables.

9. Place in oven and bake for 15-20 minutes.

4. BUCKWHEAT & VEGGIE STIRFRY

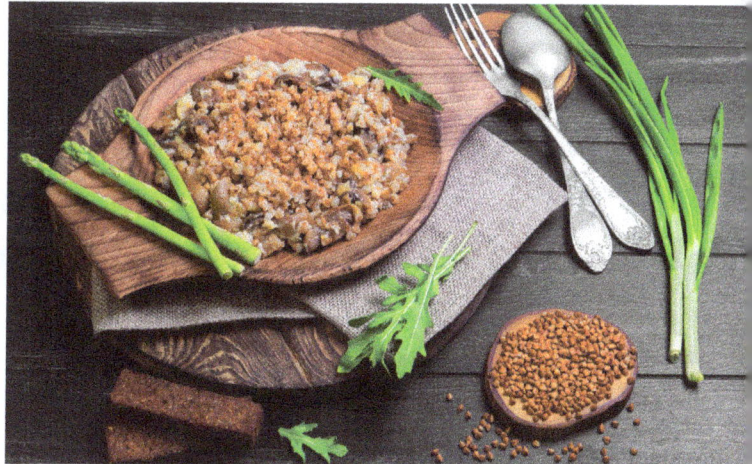 15 Minutes

Ingredients:

¼ Whole Eggplant

2 Crimini Mushrooms

2 Scallions

¼ Cups Sliced Tomatoes

½ Cup Buckwheat

Olive Oil

Cayenne, Salt & Pepper

Directions:

Stir-Fry:

1. Wash and slice all vegetables. Set aside scallions for later use.

2. Pour olive oil liberally into pan and allow to heat up.

3. Place vegetables into pan in the following order (waiting 1-2 minutes before adding the next): Eggplant, mushrooms, tomatoes.

4. Add cayenne, salt, and pepper as desired.

5. Mix the contents of the pan as you cook.

6. Cook for 8-10 minutes or until eggplant is soft and cooked through.

Buckwheat:

1. Bring 3/4 cups of water to a boil. Add buckwheat.

2. Stir while cooking for 5 minutes.

3. After 5 minutes, slide pot away from heated portion of stovepot and continue stirring progressively until all the water has been absorbed (this should take another 5 minutes).

5. SPICY LENTIL & QUINOA SOUP

15 Minutes

Ingredients:

½ Cup Lentils

¼ Cup Quinoa

2 Tbsp. of Olive Oil

¼ Yellow Onion

1/2 Tomatoes

Ginger

Cardamom, Coriander & Cayenne

Salt & Pepper

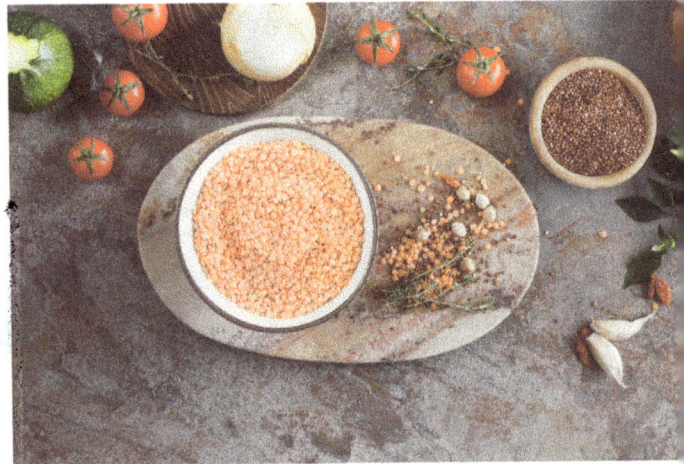

Directions:

1. Heat up a deep pan on the stovetop and add olive oil.

2. Add diced onion and allow to brown.

3. After about 5 minutes add sliced red tomato and stir.

4. After 3-4 more minutes pour in 4 cups of water and bring the mixture to a boil.

5. Stir in lentils.

6. Next stir in the quinoa.

7. Allow to cook for about 10-12 minutes until the mixture becomes a dense consistency.

8. If you would like a more watery soup, add an extra cup of water (or however much you need to get the consistency you prefer).

6. CABBAGE, RADISH & TOMATO SALAD

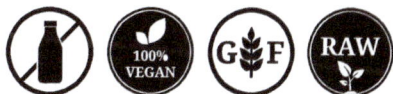

⏱ 5 Minutes

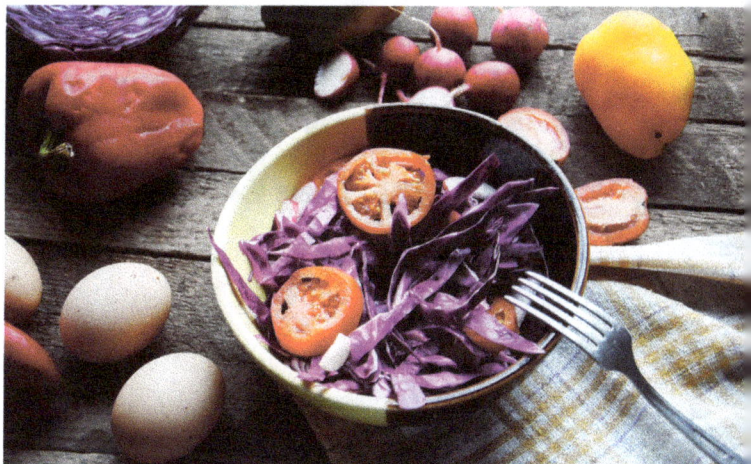

Ingredients:

1/8 Medium Cabbage

½ Tomato

¼ Red Onion

2-3 Radishes

1 tbsp. Olive Oil

Directions:

1. Wash and thinly slice cabbage.

2. Wash and chop up tomato, red onion and radishes.

3. Mix in salad bowl.

4. Add olive oil and balsamic vinegar.

LEAN BODY DINNER RECIPES

1. BAKED HADDOCK WITH PEPPERS

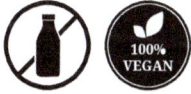

20 Minutes

Ingredients:

1/3 lb. Haddock
¼ Red Pepper
¼ Yellow Pepper
Olive Oil
Cayenne
Salt & Pepper

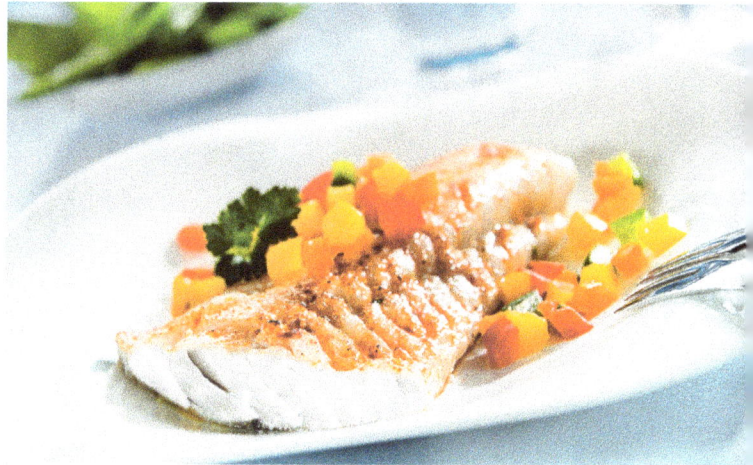

Directions:

1. Preheat oven to 400 degrees.

2. Wash and chop up peppers.

3. Cover baking dish in olive oil. Use brush to be consistent.

4. Place vegetables into baking dish.

5. Place haddock into baking dish.

6. Drizzle with olive oil.

7. Add cayenne, salt, and pepper to taste.

8. Bake for 15-20 minutes.

2. BUCKWHEAT BOWL WITH FRESH TOMATO & BASIL

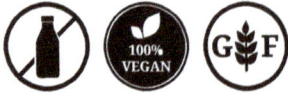

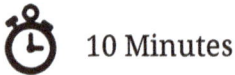 10 Minutes

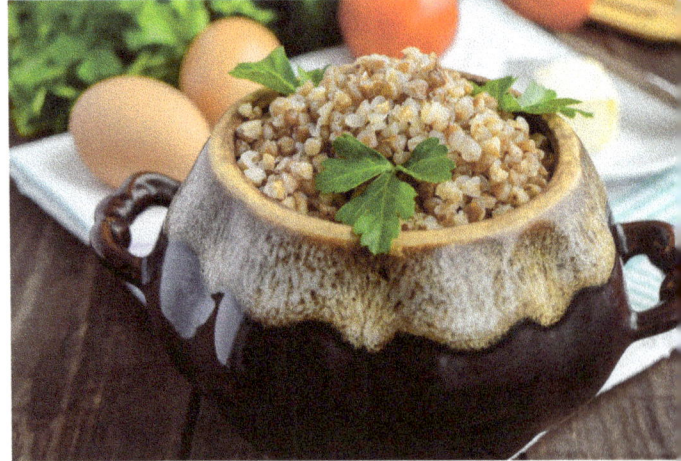

Ingredients:

½ Cup Buckwheat

¾ Heirloom Tomato

½ Avocado

Basil Leaves

Directions:

1. Bring 3/4 cups of water to a boil. Add buckwheat.

2. Stir while cooking for 5 minutes.

3. Slide pot away from the heated portion of the stoveop and continue stirring progressively until all the water has been absorbed (this should take another 5 minutes).

4. Wash and chop heirloom tomato.

5. Wash and slice avocado. Remove skin and seed.

6. Add tomato and avocado to kasha.

7. Sprinkle on basil leaves.

3. SEABASS WITH WILD RICE AND VEGETABLES

25 Minutes

Ingredients:

1/3 lb. Seabass

¼ cup Wild Rice

2 Large Slices Eggplant

1 Tomato

1 Large Carrot

Olive Oil

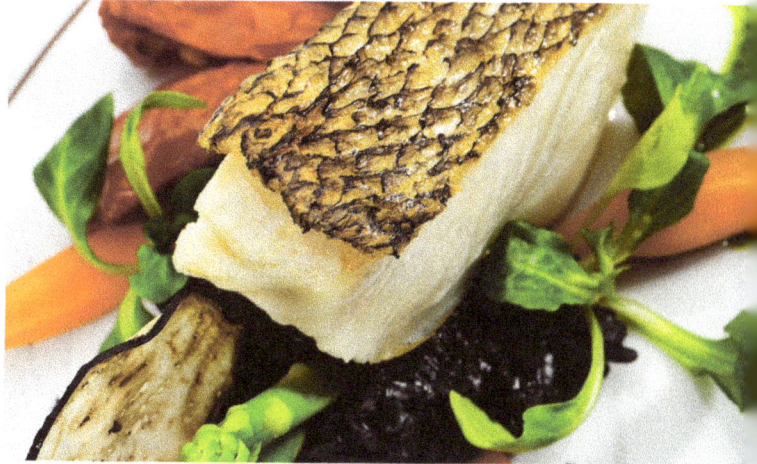

Directions:

1. Preheat oven to 450 degrees.

2. Wash eggplant, tomato and carrot.

3. Finely slice eggplant, tomato and carrot.

4. Boil ¾ cup water.

5. Place wild rice in boiling water and cook for 20 minutes.

6. Cover baking dish in olive oil. Use brush to be consistent.

7. Place chopped veggies on baking dish.

8. Place sea bass in a separate baking dish. This fish doesn't need any oil as it is incredibly oily on its own.

9. Place both dishes into oven and bake for 15-20 minutes. Fish should come out golden brown.

10. Drain any excess water from wild rice and place on dinner plate with sea-bass and vegetables.

4. PASTA WITH HOMEMADE TOMATO SAUCE

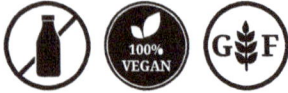

15 Minutes

Ingredients:

3 Tbsp. Olive Oil
¼ cup Brown Rice Spiral Pasta
1 Tomato
½ Red Pepper
½ Onion
Basil

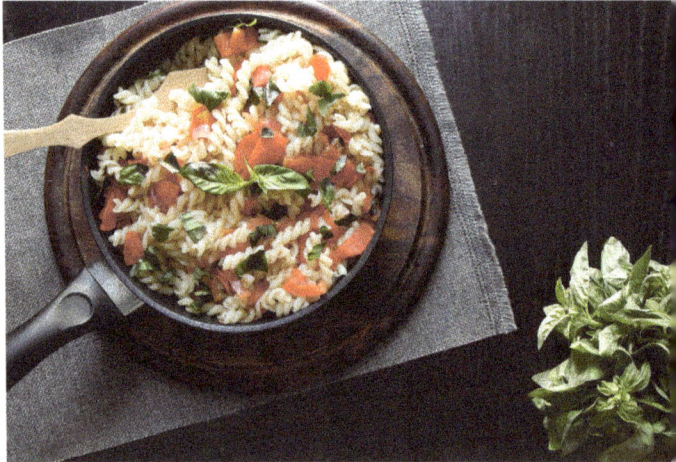

Directions:

1. Bring water to a boil.

2. Add brown rice pasta and cook for 10-12 minutes.

3. Wash tomato, red pepper and onion. Chop up finely.

4. Heat up olive oil in sauce pan.

5. Add pepper and onion first to the pan. 3-4 minutes later, add tomato.

6. Allow to simmer and cook for 5-8 minutes (while pasta is cooking).

7. Continually stir the sauce with spoon.

8. Drain pasta and place in bowl.

9. Add sauce and mix.

10. Add fresh basil.

5. ROASTED SALMON & VEGGIES

(GF) ⏱ 25 Minutes

Ingredients:

3 Tbsp. Extra Virgin Olive Oil

1/3 lb. Wild Salmon

5-6 Cherry Tomatoes

½ Onion

5-6 Brussels Sprouts

3-4 Broccoli Florets

Salt & Pepper

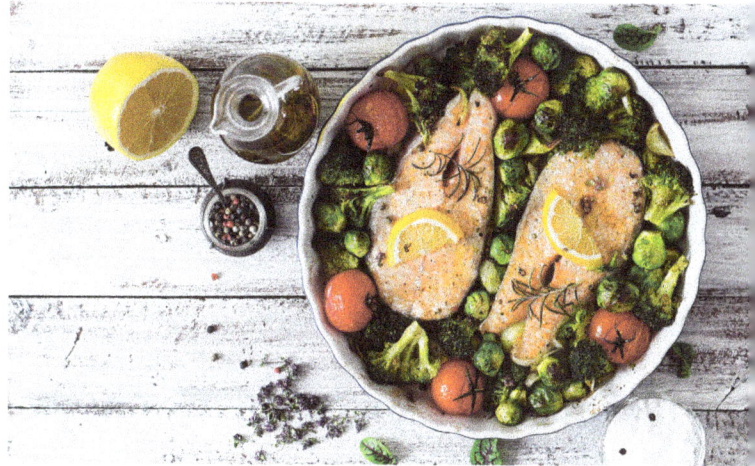

Directions:

1. Preheat oven to 450 degrees.

2. Wash tomatoes, onion, Brussels sprouts and broccoli.

3. Half the tomatoes and Brussels sprouts. Chop the onion into small pieces.

4. Add 1 tbsp. of olive oil to a ceramic baking dish. Use a brush to spread oil across entire dish.

5. Place vegetables into baking dish.

6. Drizzle with 1 tbsp. olive oil.

7. Bake vegetables for 10 minutes.

8. Prep salmon with salt & pepper to taste.

9. After 10 minutes, stir vegetables and add salmon onto baking dish.

10. Bake for another 10- 15 minutes or until salmon is cooked to your preference. The vegetables should come out golden brown.

6. BROILED SARDINES & POTATO

25 Minutes

Ingredients:

3 Tbsp. Extra Virgin Olive Oil

1-2 Sardines

1 Medium Potato

3-4 Cloves of Garlic

1 Lemon (for taste)

Dill

3-4 Sliced Olives

Salt & Pepper

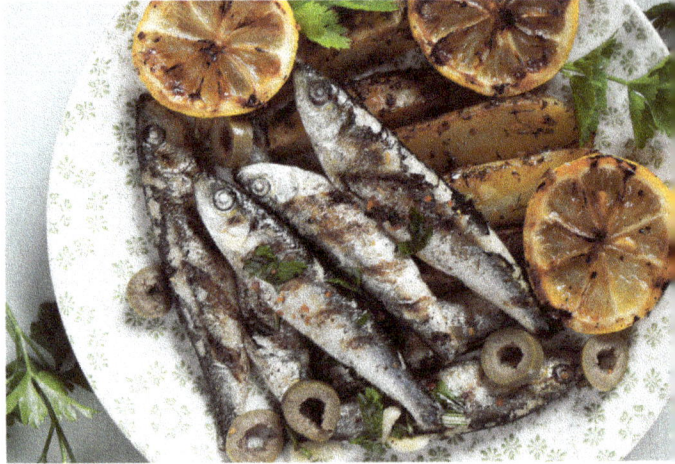

Directions:

1. Set oven to "Broil" and allow it to preheat.

2. Wash potato and cut into 1/8's.

3. Add 1 tbsp. of olive oil to a ceramic baking dish. Use brush to spread oil across entire dish.

4. Place potato slices in baking dish.

5. Add cleaned and sliced garlic on top of potato wedges.

6. Add salt and pepper.

7. Drizzle potato and garlic with 1-2 additional tablespoons of olive oil.

8. Place sardines into separate ceramic baking dish. You don't need to add oil as this fish is incredibly oily on its own.

9. If you like, add lemon slices to the sardine baking dish. You will use this lemon later on to flavor the fish as well.

10. Allow potato to broil around 20 minutes. Sardines will only need 8-10 minutes if fresh (if frozen, add 5 minutes). Flip over sardines after 5 minutes, and shuffle around potatoes after 10 minutes to get the best consistency.

11. Remove from oven and place on dinner plate.

12. Add sliced olives and dill.

13. Drizzle with more olive oil if you need.

LEAN BODY DESSERT RECIPES

1. DRIED FRUIT & NUTS

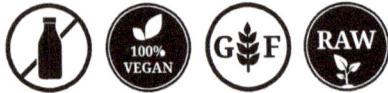

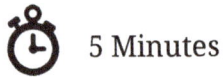 5 Minutes

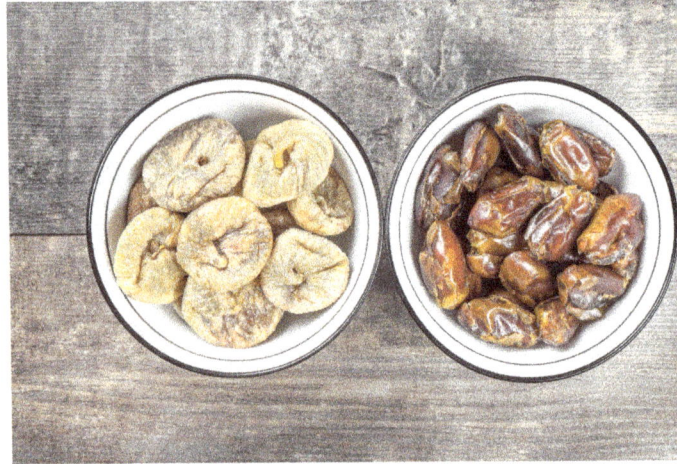

Ingredients:

1-2 Dried Turkish Figs

1-2 Dried Medjool Dates

2-4 Brazil Nuts

Directions:

1. Pull apart the figs and dates into half pieces. Remove the pits of the dates.

2. Place Brazil nut into each half of the dried fruit and enjoy.

2. STUFFED BAKED APPLES

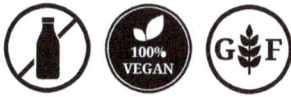

20 Minutes

Ingredients:

1 Large Fuji Apple
¼ Ripened Banana
1/8 cup Walnuts
¼ cup Previously Cooked Oatmeal
1 ½ Tbsp. Organic Maple Syrup
Cinnamon

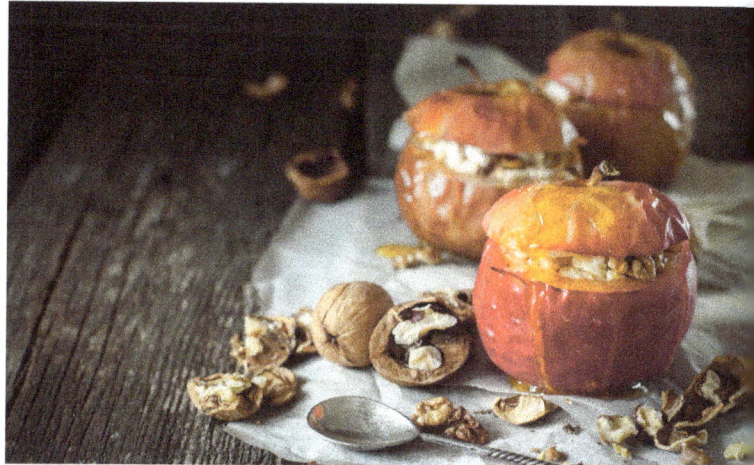

Directions:

1. Preheat oven to 400 degrees.

2. Mush up banana.

3. Chop up walnuts finely.

4. Mix ½ tbsp. maple syrup, cinnamon, banana and walnuts into previously cooked oatmeal.

5. Cut off top ¼ of apple. Remove core of the apple and keep the top quarter to replace later.

6. Pour ½ tbsp. maple syrup into the cored apple.

7. Stuff with oatmeal mixture.

8. Pour ¼ tbsp. maple syrup on top of stuffed apple and sprinkle on some more cinnamon.

9. Return the top quarter of the apple and drizzle remaining maple syrup all over the covered apple.

10. Bake for 15 minutes or until apple and oatmeal are golden brown.

3. FRO-NANA POPS

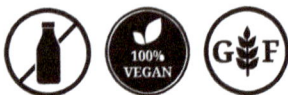

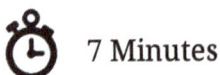

7 Minutes

Ingredients:

1/3 bar 85% Cacao Dark Chocolate

1 Large Banana Cut Into 6 Pieces (Previously Frozen)

¼ cup Chopped Walnuts

¼ cup Chopped Almonds

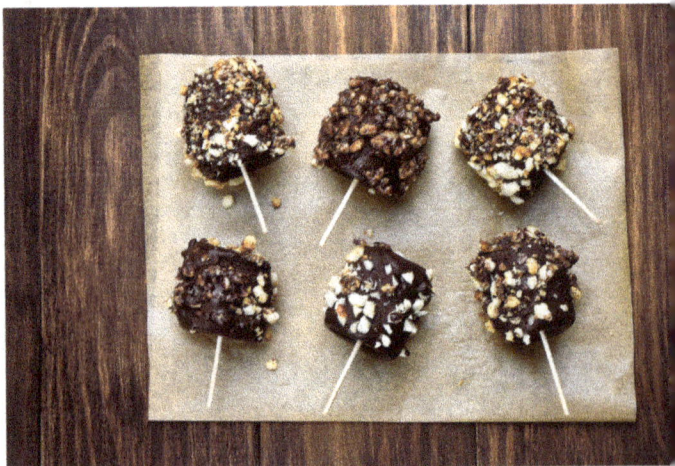

Directions:

1. Bring 1/8 cup water to a boil in a small pot.

2. Put dark chocolate into boiling water and allow it to melt. Stir occasionally.

3. Remove frozen banana chunks from freezer and place toothpicks into one end of banana like a popsicle.

4. Dip banana chunks into dark chocolate, covering entire piece.

5. Sprinkle each chocolate covered piece with walnuts, almonds or a mix of the two.

6. Allow to cool momentarily and enjoy!

7. Alternatively: Do steps 1-6 with a fresh banana. Then place on wax paper in a freezer safe container and store in freezer overnight. Enjoy when you're ready!

4. FRESH BERRIES

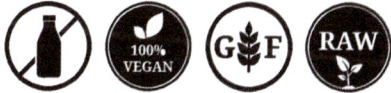

⏱ 5 Minutes

Ingredients:
Your choice of fresh berries.

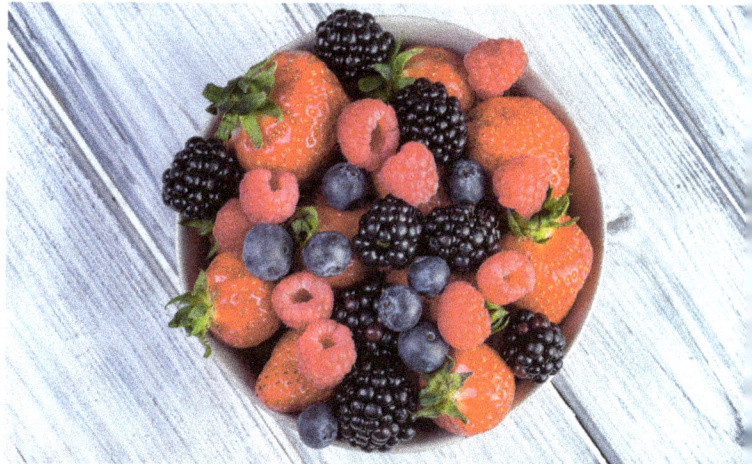

Directions:
1. Wash berries well and place in a bowl.

LEAN BODY
SNACKS

1. NUTS & DARK CHOCOLATE

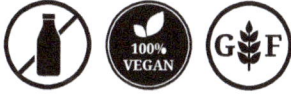

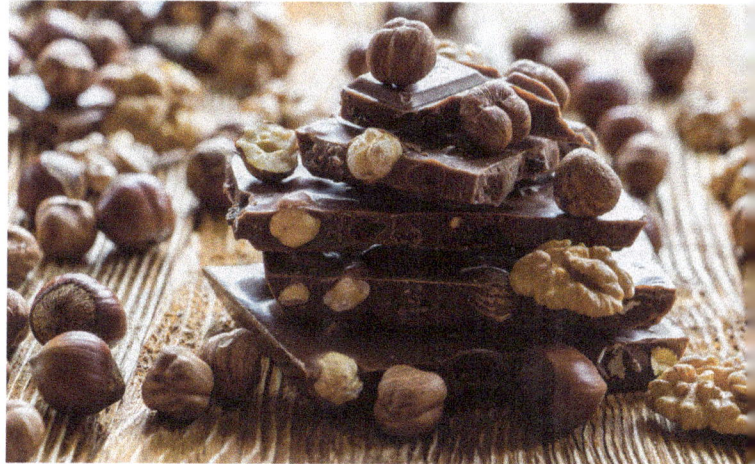

🕐 5 Minutes

Ingredients:

¼ of 85% Cacao Dark
Chocolate Bar

3-4 Hazelnuts

3-4 Walnuts

3-4 Almonds

Directions:

1. Mix and enjoy.

2. AVOCADO & VEGGIES

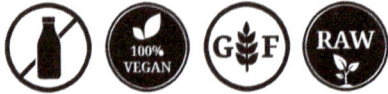

⏱ 5 Minutes

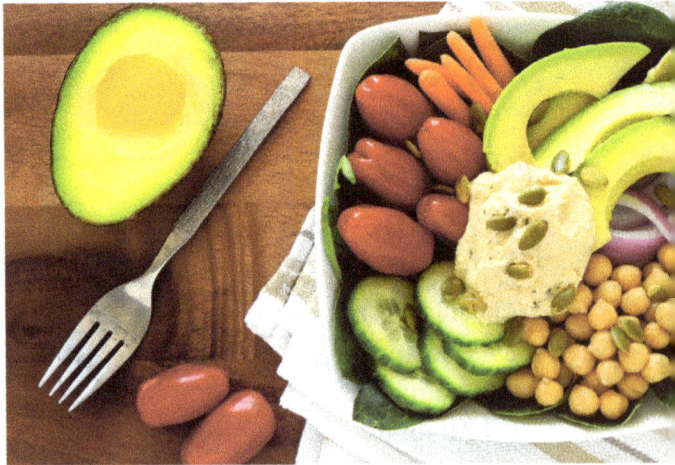

Ingredients:

½ Avocado

¼ Cucumber

4-5 Cherry Tomatoes

4-5 Carrots

Salt & Pepper

Directions:

1. Wash all of the vegetables thoroughly.

2. Wash and cut avocado in half.

3. Slice up vegetables into bite sized pieces.

4. Salt and pepper avocado and veggies to taste.

5. Scoop out avocado from shell with veggies as a "dip."

6. Alternatively, slice up avocado and eat with veggies.

3. FRESH BERRY BOWL

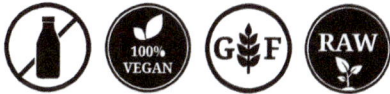

🕐 5 Minutes

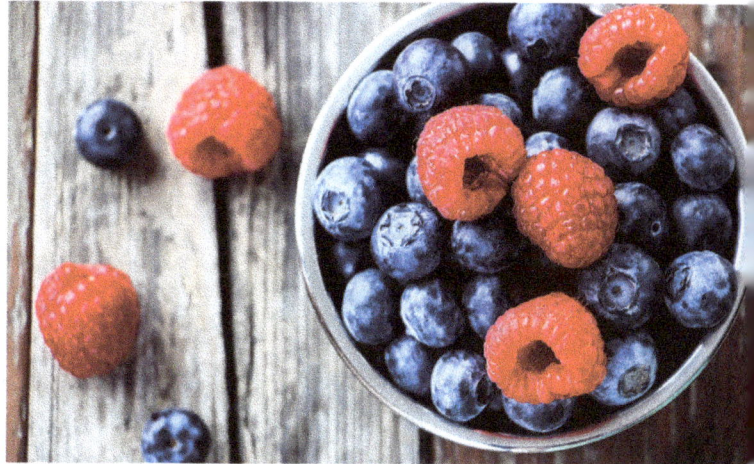

Ingredients:

¼ cup Blueberries

¼ cup Raspberries

¼ cup Blackberries

3-4 large Strawberries

Directions:

1. Wash berries well and place in a bowl.

4. FRESH VEGGIES

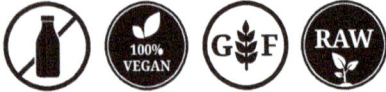

⏱ 5 Minutes

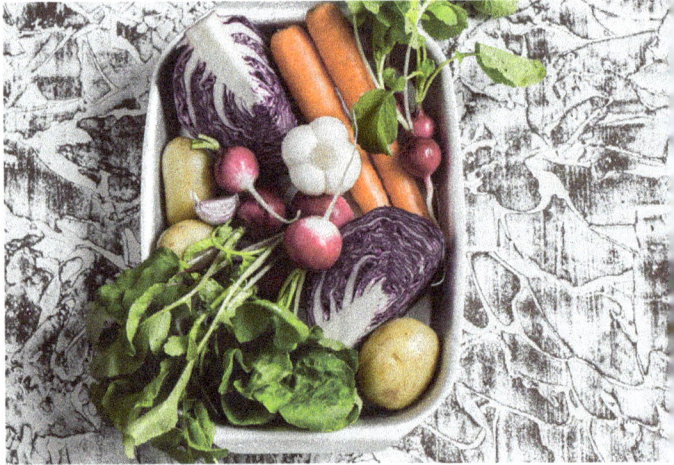

Ingredients:

1-2 Radishes

½ Large Carrot

¼ Small Cabbage

Salt & Pepper

Directions:

1. Wash and chop up vegetables.

2. Salt & Pepper to taste.

THE LEAN BODY
GROCERY LIST

Lean Body Grocery List

Below is a complete grocery list for the Lean Body Breakfast, Lunch, Dinner, Dessert, and Snack Recipes. Stock your kitchen with these ingredients so you never stray from your lean body diet.

FRUIT
- Strawberries
- Blueberries
- Raspberries
- Blackberries
- Fuji Apples
- Bananas
- Avocado
- Lemon

VEGETABLES
- Beet
- Ginger
- Brocolli
- Chard
- Romaine
- Lettuce
- Radishes
- Cherry Tomatoes
- Yellow Onions
- Red Cabbage
- Sweet Potato
- Potato
- Carrots
- Squash
- Portobello Mushroom Caps
- Red Pepper
- Yellow Pepper
- Zucchini
- Eggplant
- Crimini Mushrooms
- Scallions
- Red Onion
- Cucumber
- Heirloom Tomato
- Basil
- Brussel Sprouts
- Garlic
- Dill

GRAINS

- Steel Cut Oatmeal
- Buckwheat Flour
- Rye Bread
- Buckwheat
- Lentils
- Quinoa
- Wild Rice
- Brown Rice Pasta

FISH

- Cod
- Haddock
- Seabass
- Salmon
- Sardines

BULK

- Dried Dates
- Dried Apricots
- Dried Figs
- Raisins
- Walnuts
- Hazelnuts
- Almonds

ADDITIONAL INGREDIENTS

- Apple Sauce
- Baking Soda
- First Cold Pressed Olive Oil
- Maple Syrup
- Balsamic Vinegar
- Cayenne Pepper
- Cumin
- Cardamom
- Coriander
- Cinnamon
- Salt & Pepper
- 85% Cacao Dark Chocolate

THE
4-WEEK
LEAN BODY
MEAL PLAN

The 4-Week Lean Body Meal Plan

Week 1		
Monday	Breakfast	Fruit Jam on Toast
	Lunch	Stuffed Mushrooms
	Dinner	Buckwheat Bowl with Fresh Tomato & Basil
Tuesday	Breakfast	Buckwheat Pancakes
	Lunch	Spicy Lentil & Quinoa Soup
	Dinner	Baked Haddock with Peppers
Wednesday	Breakfast	Breakfast Toast
	Lunch	Fresh Vegetable Salad
	Dinner	Roasted Salmon & Veggies
Thursday	Breakfast	Oatmeal and Fresh Fruit
	Lunch	Buckwheat & Veggie Stirfry
	Dinner	Pasta with Homemade Tomato Sauce
Friday	Breakfast	Buckwheat Pancakes
	Lunch	Cabbage, Radish, & Tomato Salad
	Dinner	Broiled Sardines & Potato
Saturday	Breakfast	Oatmeal with Walnuts/Berries/Cinnamon
	Lunch	Baked Cod & Veggies
	Dinner	Buckwheat Bowl with Fresh Tomato & Basil
Sunday	Breakfast	Beet Smoothie
	Lunch	Spicy Lentil & Quinoa Soup
	Dinner	Seabass with Wild Rice & Vegetables

Week 2		
Monday	Breakfast	Oatmeal and Fresh Fruit
	Lunch	Cabbage, Radish, & Tomato Salad
	Dinner	Roasted Salmon & Veggies
Tuesday	Breakfast	Fruit Jam on Toast
	Lunch	Buckwheat & Veggie Stirfry
	Dinner	Pasta with Homemade Tomato Sauce
Wednesday	Breakfast	Oatmeal with Walnuts/Berries/Cinnamon
	Lunch	Stuffed Mushrooms
	Dinner	Baked Haddock with Peppers
Thursday	Breakfast	Buckwheat Pancakes
	Lunch	Fresh Vegetable Salad
	Dinner	Broiled Sardines & Potato
Friday	Breakfast	Breakfast Toast
	Lunch	Baked Cod & Veggies
	Dinner	Seabass with Wild Rice & Vegetables
Saturday	Breakfast	Oatmeal with Walnuts/Berries/Cinnamon
	Lunch	Spicy Lentil & Quinoa Soup
	Dinner	Buckwheat Bowl with Fresh Tomato & Basil
Sunday	Breakfast	Piece of Fruit: Apple or Banana
	Lunch	Fresh Vegetable Salad
	Dinner	Pasta with Homemade Tomato Sauce

Week 3		
Monday	Breakfast	Buckwheat Pancakes
	Lunch	Baked Cod & Veggies
	Dinner	Roasted Salmon & Veggies
Tuesday	Breakfast	Breakfast Toast
	Lunch	Spicy Lentil & Quinoa Soup
	Dinner	Buckwheat Bowl with Fresh Tomato & Basil
Wednesday	Breakfast	Oatmeal with Walnuts/Berries/Cinnamon
	Lunch	Cabbage, Radish, & Tomato Salad
	Dinner	Broiled Sardines & Potato
Thursday	Breakfast	Fruit Jam on Toast
	Lunch	Fresh Vegetable Salad
	Dinner	Baked Haddock with Peppers
Friday	Breakfast	Oatmeal and Fresh Fruit
	Lunch	Buckwheat & Veggie Stirfry
	Dinner	Pasta with Homemade Tomato Sauce
Saturday	Breakfast	Fruit Jam on Toast
	Lunch	Stuffed Mushrooms
	Dinner	Roasted Salmon & Veggies
Sunday	Breakfast	Beet Smoothie
	Lunch	Cabbage, Radish, & Tomato Salad
	Dinner	Seabass with Wild Rice & Vegetables

Week 4		
Monday	Breakfast	Breakfast Toast
	Lunch	Buckwheat & Veggie Stirfry
	Dinner	Pasta with Homemade Tomato Sauce
Tuesday	Breakfast	Oatmeal with Walnuts/Berries/Cinnamon
	Lunch	Stuffed Mushrooms
	Dinner	Roasted Salmon & Veggies
Wednesday	Breakfast	Oatmeal and Fresh Fruit
	Lunch	Fresh Vegetable Salad
	Dinner	Buckwheat Bowl with Fresh Tomato & Basil
Thursday	Breakfast	Breakfast Toast
	Lunch	Baked Cod & Veggies
	Dinner	Seabass with Wild Rice & Vegetables
Friday	Breakfast	Buckwheat Pancakes
	Lunch	Spicy Lentil & Quinoa Soup
	Dinner	Baked Haddock with Peppers
Saturday	Breakfast	Fruit Jam on Toast
	Lunch	Cabbage, Radish, & Tomato Salad
	Dinner	Broiled Sardines & Potato
Sunday	Breakfast	Piece of Fruit: Apple or Banana
	Lunch	Baked Cod & Veggies
	Dinner	Pasta with Homemade Tomato Sauce

TESTIMONIALS

Lashawn

Age: 25

Weight Lost: 105 Pounds

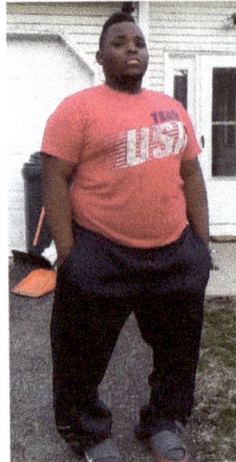

Before

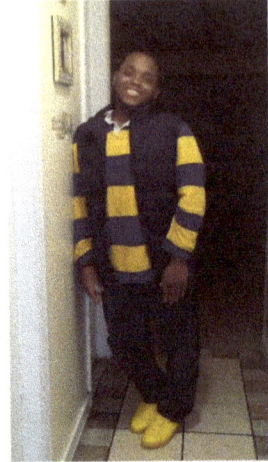

After

"I started this weight loss journey after feeling tired of being overweight and having knee pain. At 23 I began working out more than usual and cutting back on all the junk food. I started the weight loss journey at 295 lbs. and from the hard work I am now at 190 lbs. I began meal prepping and eating lean. Steaming vegetables from the farmers market has become sort of my thing. I began running 1 mile and a half and then walking out the remainder back home. I play tennis 3 times a week for about 2 and a half hours. I learned that going for a walk or slight jog after every meal gives you strength. Another thing that was important on my journey was not eating after 8. Cutting back completely on the wine and alcohol even socially got me to the point where I barely drink it any more. I stopped drinking soda completely and made water my best friend. It's the simple things that result in the biggest weight loss."

Alex

Age: 33
Weight Lost: 27 Pounds

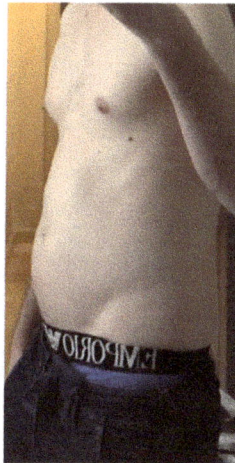
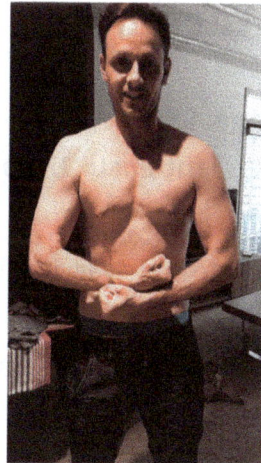

Before   **After**

"I started to drink water only, cutting out sugary drinks in particular. I stopped going to fast food chains and eating fried food, limited my red meat to once every two weeks, and stopped eating out at restaurants more generally. I stopped eating dairy products and restricted my wheat intake. Also, I started eating lean protein mainly—chicken breast, tuna, and other fish. My weight dropped from 182 to 155. I feel leaner, less bloated, and more energized. For my workouts, I was a college tennis player and so I started playing tennis again more regularly and with more intensity. Before, I would just come out and hit some balls in a recreational way, but I've found other high level players to hit with and play sets. I'm running a bit more (didn't do any running before) and recently started lifting weights. Also—I allow myself one cheat meal each week."

Adrian

Age: 29
Weight Lost: 12 Pounds

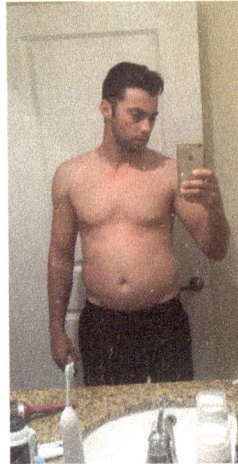 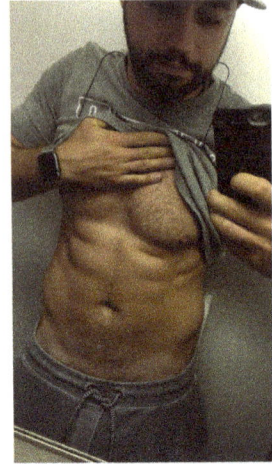

Before   **After**

"Before I was hardly doing any cardio at all and when I did work out, it would pretty much always be weights. Once I started doing a cardio-based workout, the lean body took form. I stopped drinking too—only one day a week, which helped a lot. Also, I would have a solid lunch and dinner but not eat very much for breakfast. Between meals I would feel some hunger and maybe snack on an apple—but I would usually hold off on eating until the next meal. That part was huge—enjoying a full meal (and feeling satiated) but not eating between sit-downs so I wasn't taking in any extra calories."

Pri

Age: 29
Weight Lost: 14 Pounds

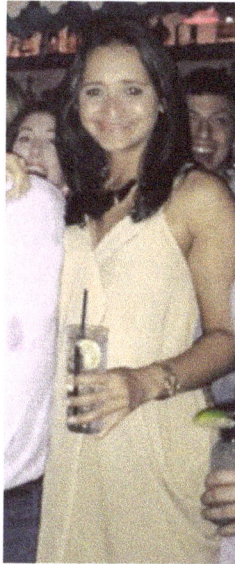
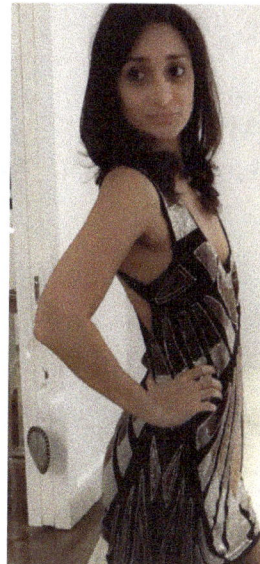

Before   **After**

"Once I started to cut out unhealthy food and pay attention to what I was eating, the results came. I regulated portion size, dairy intake, and focused in particular on what I was eating during the week. A few years ago, I used to eat pretty poorly. Bascially anything I could get my hands on whether it was pizza, sandwiches, bacon egg and cheese, you name it. Stress eating mainly. At my last job (Goldman Sachs), we would be given $25 to spend for dinner, so people went nuts and took full advantage of ordering hefty meals. I now have a clear-cut routine: banana and green tea for breakfast, salad for lunch, and I give myself flexiblity in terms of what I eat for dinner. I also started working out more rigorously, more cardio and muscle toning. I limit my alcohol intake to 1-2 times per week. I don't like drinking during the week because it messes up my workout schedule. At one point at Goldman I think I weighed 126 and now I'm 112/113. I feel much lighter and energetic and more confident about myself and body and overall well-being and level of happiness. "

Lyuda

Age: 29
Weight Lost: 15 Pounds

"I used to diet and exercise. Now I eat and train. This mindset shift has made all the difference and I would have never been able to adopt it without Jon's guidance. I literally did not eat 1 gram of carbs for years and was starved and constantly depleted of energy. When I did eat, I ate diet products, including diet soda (Orange Crush was my favorite). Even if I didn't have energy, I would

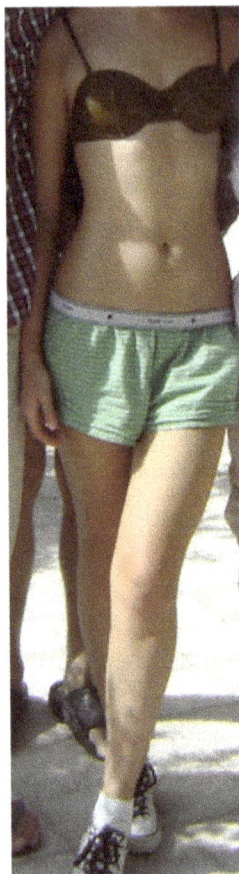 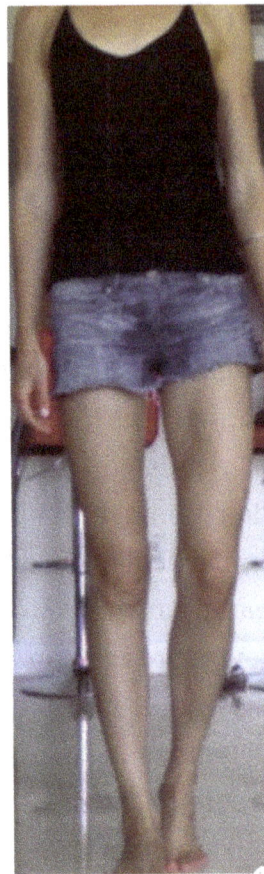

Before   **After**

still go to the gym and do 2 hours on the elliptical machine. My habits were unhealthy. I was never comfortable in my skin. And looking back now, I can't believe I consumed these nutrition-less products and then expected my body to perform in a workout later on. I still feel guilty about how badly I mistreated my body.

With Jon, I learned a holistic approach to health. I started to eat nutritious foods and after a few months (and pounds lost) I started to believe that you can actually eat well AND look good. I always eat to satiation, often enjoy dessert, and have so much energy to work out powerfully and still be able to focus and concentrate on my work throughout the day. I truly think of myself as an athlete now, something I never even considered before. I work out hard to get my body to perform at its best and make sure to fuel it with nutritious food.

I only focus on the nutrition in my food now and do not worry about calories. Because I am in tune with my body (and it is not going haywire due to crazy chemicals from diet products) I can trust my instincts in terms of hunger and satiation. I never experience the cravings that I used to. It has been 5 years since my lifestyle has changed and staying committed with a consistent program has worked wonders. I'm down from 137 to 122lbs and feel light, fit, lean and most of all happy! Every workout is exciting because I am always training to progress—to run faster. And knowing how to cook and make my own meals has freed me from worrying about calories.

Now that I know what being healthy and vibrant feels like, I will never live any other way. Just try this program and you will feel the same!"

Ethan

Age: 18

High School Soccer Player. Improved Fitness, Diet, and Lifestyle

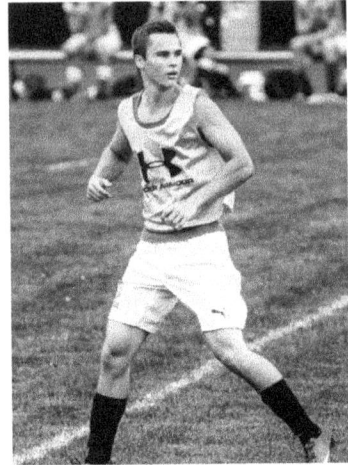

"From my personal experience the advice was amazing, I cannot say enough good things about it. At the start of the process not going to lie it was difficult and I didn't think I could do it. After I kept sticking with everything, it became a smoother transition to becoming healthier and staying fit. I started right before I was going to try out for my high school soccer team. As a senior I wanted it to be a year to remember. Thanks to the program, eating healthier became a big part of my success. The healthy food made me feel extremely better and made me have more energy which led to me playing one of my best seasons that I could remember. After soccer I still kept with my diet and kept with the activities that were keeping me fit and healthy. Throughout the year I felt amazing, which also led to many positive things in my senior year such as getting better grades than usual and just being in a better and positive mood."

Matt

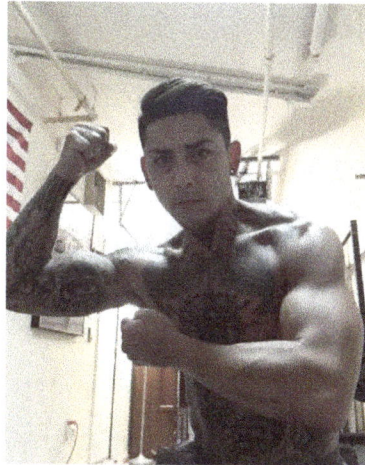

Age: 35
Weight Lost: 20 Pounds

"The big changes came once I started wearing sweats during my workouts and shifting my training to more cardio. Before, I was working out only in the gym, but then began running outside and the weight started to melt off. Also, steaming vegetables was huge for me. Jon showed me the steaming basket and how to steam vegetables on the stovetop—something I hadn't done before. I started cooking quinoa and bringing steamed veggies with quinoa and grilled chicken to work for lunch. Also, I cut back on drinking. I used to have a few beers a night during the week and even more on the weekends. Now, I don't drink at all during the week and have a lot less when I do go out. All of this combined got me lean and healthy. The program works and I recommend it! It's about small changes, but small changes add up and they have helped me in living a healthier, focused, fit, and optimized life."

John

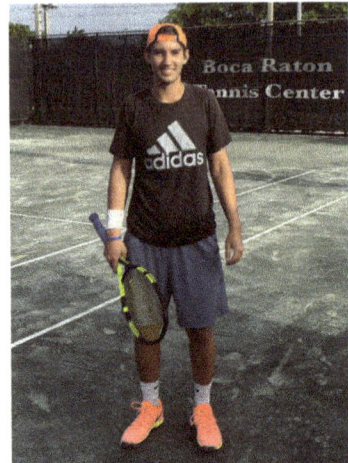

Age: 19

Weight Lost: 15 Pounds

College Tennis Player. Improved Fitness and Sports Performance

"Since beginning the lean lifestyle, I have noticed major improvements in my physical ability. I have worked my way into much better shape, shredding 15 pounds since starting this program. I move much better on the tennis court and have become extremely confident in my athletic performance. It is not easy, but it is worth it."

Larry

Age: 61
Weight Lost: 20 Pounds

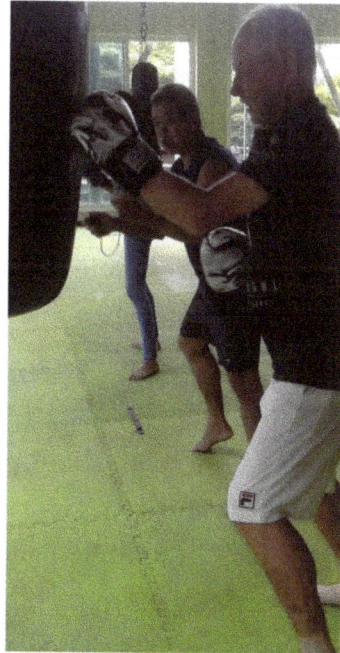

"I met Jon about 18 months ago at a tennis event and we got to talking. He explained his approach to life and I was very interested and he later offered to send me a preliminary copy of his book. After reading it, I decided to change my life in many ways. Getting into great physical shape, and getting lean. Using my sports background in tennis and muay thai boxing to become fitter and stronger. Making physical training and a healthy diet a part of my life. I am now leaner, in great shape and smarter. I used to drink a few sodas every day. I haven't had a Dr. Pepper, Coke, etc. in months and months and months. All because of Jon's way of life that I embraced. My son Danny is a tennis player too and I have gotten him to follow many of the lean body tips. We're planning to play father and son doubles tournaments, which will be a great way to keep healthy, stay in shape, and have a lot of fun at the same time."

Jon (Author)

Age: 28
Weight Lost: 20 Pounds

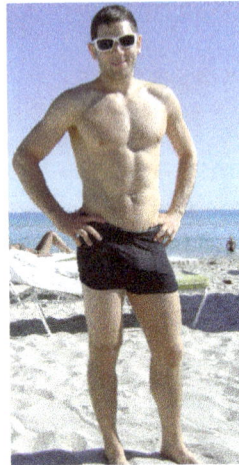 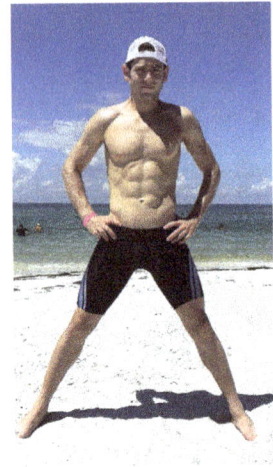

Before   **After**

"When I competed as a college tennis player, I was completely absorbed by the weightlifting culture. I was strong, but way too heavy and my body wasn't working efficiently. I hadn't mastered my nutrition or the routines necessary to build and sustain the lean body. Over the course of the last five years (two of which I competed on the pro tennis tour), I started to understand that the lean body was the gateway to performing at my peak on the tennis court—and feeling my best overall in life. The secrets, tricks, routines, and advice presented in the The Lean Body Manual took nearly a decade to develop. My passion for fitness, nutrition, and sports performance, and my unrelenting drive to figure all of this out, has led me to develop this unique and sustainable approach to building a fit, lean, enduring, and healthy body. The strategies I present here will allow you to circumvent all of the noise in the modern fitness and diet industry, and emerge on the other side with a clear-cut plan of action—one that will transform your way of thinking and approach to fitness, diet, and health...for life. I am excited to present this to you and hope you will benefit from the lean body program as much as I have."

Elliot

Age: 29

Improved Fitness, Health, Diet, Quality of Life, and Decreased Pain

"After having the chance to learn from Jon about his approach to fitness and nutrition, I shifted my views on what being healthy really entails. It was not that I was relatively overweight or consuming terrible foods. Before, I was primarily focused on building and maintaining muscles and fueling this with decent foods, admittedly too much consumption of animal products. However, I was often in much pain.

My focus changed to workouts for a more sustainable life for the long term (cardio, body weight training and stretching) and foods, notably more whole foods and less animal products, to nourish the body and mind. Basically supporting a more natural body to be able to live generally better and in less pain."

Charles

Age: 69

Weight Lost: 120 Pounds

"So I met Jon and his fiancé at a function and was awe struck by what great shape both were in. What got me truly inspired was when I started seeing their food preparation featured on their blog. To see what painstaking attention they take in the preparation, the balance of ying and yang, the selection of ingredients and the rationale towards preparing their meals or what one would deem fuel to energize their bodies was eye opening. Being a 124lbs (at that time) overweight, I decided to take life lengthening action. I decided that I would propagate Jon's attitude towards food and exercise. Fast forward two years. Today I am down 120lbs (actually more, but muscle weighs more than fat)— from 354lbs I am now a svelte, well-built 230lbs. Today food is my body's energy, the energy I use to fuel my daily 2 hour workouts.

I encourage everyone to make changes for the better and I encourage you to read the good word of Jon Pearlman, a fit-for-life coach."

Jonathan

Age: 35

Former Top-Ranked Tennis Player Getting Back into Shape

"I started running and playing tennis in the sweatsuit, trying to sweat as much as possible. I focused on eating healthier and also when and how much I was eating during the day. The only times I would eat would be breakfast, lunch, dinner, and one snack during the day. Four times and that was it. No munching. Restricting the eating combined with the cardio workouts in the sweatsuit got me the results. Also, I only drank water, nothing else. That was key."

Morcene

Age: 56
Weight Lost: 20 Pounds

"Living a great life is all about lifestyle. Just by chance I was asked to try a few recipes by a guy named Jon Pearlman. I was blown away— not only did the food taste good but I found myself with more energy and shedding some weight. Jon Pearlman has a "Plan" that motivates you to eat well and stay in shape. It really works! I've lived it for 14 months and I've lost 20 pounds and am keeping it off. I feel and look great, you would never guess my age."

Olga

Age: 30
Weight Lost: 18 Pounds

"Jon's lean body approach awakened me to fact that in my busy life I lost a sense of nourishment and the movement my body needed and deserved. Before starting the regimen I was always dieting and exercising merely to damage control my splurges. I dreaded counting calories and spending hours on cardio machines at the gym. The whole process felt exhausting to the point that I couldn't enjoy my life anymore.

After changing my diet to eat the wholesome, primarily plant based foods the lean body approach advises, I immediately felt a surge in energy. My body felt lighter and my cravings for 'cheat foods' subsided. I started to view exercise as training and shorter bursts of it left me filled with endorphins. Instead of craving cupcakes I was craving the energy boost of a timed run. After I realized how much better my body functioned I was hooked and the results followed naturally as my body transformed into the athletic and lean physique that it was always intended to be."

Mesa

Age: 25

Former College Tennis Player.
Optimized Approach to Sports and Life

"I discovered Jon's blog 'Creating Substance' early on and the daily blog posts were a constant motivator and reminder of what it takes to be lean. Although a tennis player my whole life, I was not always aware of the hard work required to truly be an athlete. And that is what is so special about Jon's approach to fitness and nutrition—it isn't about being a world class sportsman with god-given talent, it is about getting the most out of your body in a way that every single person can as long as they remain disciplined. The framework is simple and can be applied by anyone willing to make it work. You just need to buy into the message and get over the fact that it might be out of the ordinary and seem a bit over the top at first. Upon further reflection, it should be apparent that it only ever seemed that way compared to what has unfortunately become the norm today."

Hamid

Age: 34
Weight Lost: 10 Pounds

"I focused on controlling what I was eating by preparing my own food. Before, I wasn't paying much attention to my diet and would eat microwavable burritos from the gas station on the go. I started taking a prepared lunch with me every day to work. This alone would have been enough to get me results, but I didn't stop there. Based on Jon's advice, I put care into the exact type of fuel I was giving my body. Lots of veggies and fish. Less cheese and fattening ad-ons. No carbs after 6pm. I'm feeling lighter, healthier, more energized, and sharper mentally. Jon's lean body approach is incredibly effective and I would highly recommend it!"

Max

Age: 28

Improved Health, Fitness, and Lifestyle

"Following a weekly exercise plan/schedule has made staying fit much easier. Instead of deciding each day if/when I'm going to work out, I plan out my week and know what I'll be doing well in advance. The same goes for meals: when I plan my meals in advance and have healthy ingredients stocked and ready to be prepared, I find no reason to spend money on unhealthy fast food. I've found that planning ahead with respect to fitness and nutrition makes living a healthy lifestyle a lot easier."

Takura

Age: 27

Healthier Lifestyle and Improved Eating Habits

"I have definitely changed my nutrition. I have cut out red meat, no eating after late hours and I only take in carbohydrates before my planned workouts so I can use that as fuel to be burnt. I have also become more conscious of eating vegetables and fruits everyday. So instead of eating a cookie, I try to replace that with something highly nutritious and healthier such as fruit."

Dave

Age: 58
Weight Lost: 30 Pounds

"I asked my friend who is over 50 what her secret was to looking so youthful. She said I'm on the Jon Pearlman Plan, and I said what's that—what's the Jon Pearlman Plan. She said, well it's a complete lifestyle change—Jon Pearlman says you have to be aware of what you eat and you have to exercise and he has a specific formula for combining the two. She really did look good so I got some of the recipes from the Jon Pearlmam Plan and I started eating well, running 3 miles in the morning. It's been about 2 years now and I've lost 30 pounds and I've kept it off."

Ali

Age: 28

Boosted Energy and Improved Nutrition

"I cook up a big batch of grains on Sunday evening, which I eat before I leave work to fuel weekday evening workouts. The grains give me the energy I need to reach my athletic potential after a day in the office. They taste good too; my colleagues are always jealous when I take out a hot tub of healthy grains while they're forced to snack on cookies from the vending machine."

Acknowledgements

Thank you to my mom, grandma, grandfather, fiancée, and uncle, Scott. Your love, support and belief enabled me to see this project through. Without all of you behind me throughout this journey I never could have gotten there.

Thank you to my long-time coach and mentor Nandor Veres, my editor Jeremy Blachman, my coaches at Harvard, Dave Fish and Andrew Rueb, and the long list of trainers, coaches, and mentors who assisted me throughout this process: Alex Gauthier, Adrian Chermaci, Will Magee, Vince Baudat, Nandor Veres Jr., Tim Bayley, and John Termotto. The opportunity to perfect the lean body approach and complete this book came about because of a strong Feel Good Support Network, and I am grateful to all who have supported me along the way.

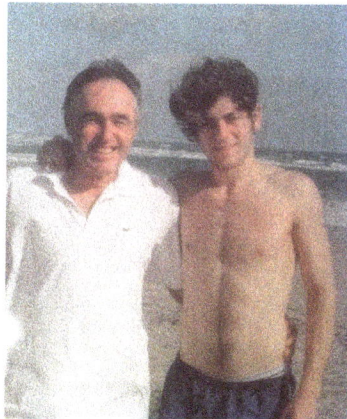

My long-time coach and mentor, Nandor Veres, educated me in the proper physical routines to achieve peak fitness and health.

About the Author

Jon Pearlman is the co-founder of Mission Lean, a digital fitness platform and app that targets lean body fitness. Download the Mission Lean app from the Apple or Google Play store and go to **www.MissionLean.com** to find out more about Mission Lean's offerings.

Jon is a former #1 singles player for the Harvard tennis team and ATP-ranked touring tennis pro. Jon's background in tennis and his passion for fitness and nutrition has made him uniquely positioned to be an advocate and ambassador for the lean body. He received his Certified Personal Trainer (CPT) and Fitness Nutrition Specialist (FNS) credentials from the American Council on Exercise. Jon lives in South Florida with his wife.